Common Problems in Pregnancy

Common Problems in Pregnancy:

An Evidence-Based Guide

By

Kassam Mahomed

Cambridge
Scholars
Publishing

Common Problems in Pregnancy: An Evidence-Based Guide

By Kassam Mahomed

This book first published 2022

Cambridge Scholars Publishing

Lady Stephenson Library, Newcastle upon Tyne, NE6 2PA, UK

British Library Cataloguing in Publication Data
A catalogue record for this book is available from the British Library

ISBN (10): 1-5275-8026-1
ISBN (13): 978-1-5275-8026-8

This book is dedicated to all the medical and midwifery staff who work constantly to provide care to women under their care; care that is based on the best available evidence.

TABLE OF CONTENTS

CHAPTER ONE

ABDOMINAL PAIN IN PREGNANCY

Gestation < 20 weeks

Need to exclude

- Miscarriage
- Pregnancy of unknown location
- Constipation
- Round ligament pain
    - pain is often bilateral and over the sides of the uterus
    - it radiates into the groin
    - it is worsened by movements like getting up from a chair/bed
- Urinary tract infection
- Fibroids
- Ovarian cyst accidents such as:
    - corpus luteum cysts
        - these cysts begin to regress after 12 weeks and are often managed expectantly
    - haemorrhage/rupture
        - women present with pain and the diagnosis is confirmed on an ultrasound scan. Pain usually settles over 24-48 hours
    - cyst torsion
        - there is sudden onset of pain which is often unilateral in the lower abdomen with associated nausea. Cysts are usually > 5cm in diameter
        - ultrasound scan is not very useful in its diagnosis
            - offer urgent laparoscopy if torsion is suspected clinically

- Bowel related
    - appendicitis
        - pain may be towards right hypochondrium at later gestation
            - CT scan is useful
            - MRI is diagnostic in almost all cases
            - appendicectomy is performed by laparoscopy in most cases
                - risk of miscarriage is low if appendix has not ruptured but may be up to 30% in first trimester if ruptured
                - preterm labour may occur in about 10% of cases if they present in the second trimester
            - do not delay surgery
    - bowel obstruction
        - this occurs mostly as a result of adhesions
            - X-ray of the abdomen in erect and supine position is usually diagnostic
            - ultrasound scan of the abdomen may also be helpful in making a diagnosis
                - consider conservative management initially
                - perform surgery as a second resort
- Pancreatitis
    - women present with severe epigastric pain radiating into the back. Pain is colicky if there are associated gall stones as well
    - serum amylase and lipase are elevated
    - gall stones are present in > 70% of cases
    - CT scan may delineate areas of necrosis
    - endoscopic retrograde cholangiopancreatography may be useful in making the diagnosis
    - consider early cholecystectomy if gall stones are present
        - offer conservative care initially
        - some recommend early aggressive surgical treatment
        - consider intensive care unit admission

- Acute cholecystitis
  - women present with colicky epigastric or right hypochondrial pain
    - aim for conservative management—especially in the first and third trimesters
    - treat with intravenous fluids, analgesia and antibiotics
      - recommend postpartum laparoscopic cholecystectomy

Recommended Reading

1. Mahomed K and Kumar S. Abdominal pain. In *High Risk Pregnancy: Management Options*. Eds. James DK, Steer PJ, Weiner CP et al. E Saunders 5th Edition 2021 pp. 1017-26.
2. Bax T, Macha M, Mayberry J. The utility of CT scan for the diagnostic evaluation of acute abdominal pain. *Am. J. Surg.* 2019 May; 217(5): 959-966.
3. Mali P. Pancreatitis in pregnancy: etiology, diagnosis, treatment, and outcomes. *Hepatobiliary & Pancreat. Dis. Int.* 2016 Aug; 15(4): 434-8.

CHAPTER TWO

ABDOMINAL TRAUMA IN PREGNANCY

Risks include placental abruption, preterm labour, massive feto-maternal haemorrhage, uterine rupture, and fetal loss which may occur even with relatively minor degrees of abdominal trauma.

With major trauma there is the risk of fractures, organ damage, hypovolaemic shock, cardiopulmonary collapse, and cardiac arrest.

Clinical presentation

- Symptoms will depend on gestational age
- Abdominal guarding and rebound tenderness may be less prominent than in non-pregnant women

Management

- First assess if the woman needs any resuscitation
- Administer Rh(D) immunoglobulin to all Rh-negative women who are > 12 weeks pregnant
- If gestational age is 20 weeks or above:
    - exclude placental abruption and preterm labour
    - assess fetal wellbeing
    - request ultrasound scan if there are any concerns
    - in rhesus negative women assess the degree of feto-maternal haemorrhage to guide dose of rhesus immunoglobulin
    - it is not recommended to perform a Kleihauer-Betke test to make or exclude a diagnosis of placental abruption
    - recommend continuous cardiotocography for at least 4 hours
        - cease after 4 hours and allow the woman to go home in cases of minor trauma if:
            - there is no abdominal pain or tenderness
            - there is no vaginal bleeding
            - cardiotocography (CTG) is normal with no uterine activity

- recommend continued observation for 24 hours if:
  - during the first 4 hours the trace is non reassuring
  - there is evidence of uterine tenderness or contractions
- admit and observe for 24 hours with intermittent continuous CTG if there is:
  - any vaginal bleeding or rupture of membranes
  - any uterine tenderness or abdominal bruising
  - presence of any uterine contractions
- recommend steroid loading if she is at risk of preterm birth < 35 weeks
- on discharge, advise her to return to hospital if:
  - there is any abdominal pain
  - she has any uterine contractions and / or vaginal bleeding
  - she has any concern about fetal movements

- In severe cases of trauma, consider a peri mortem caesarean section. This should be performed within 4 minutes of no response to effective cardiopulmonary resuscitation (CPR)

Recommended Reading

1. Huls CK, Detlefs C. Trauma in pregnancy. *Semin. Perinatol.* 2018; 42(1): 13-20.
2. Greco PS, Day LJ, Pearlman MD et al. Guidance for Evaluation and Management of Blunt Abdominal Trauma in Pregnancy. *Obstet. Gynecol.* 2019 Dec; 134(6): 1343-1357.
3. Pearce C, Martin SR. Trauma and considerations unique to pregnancy. *Obstet. Gynecol. Clin. North Am.* 2016; 43(4): 791-808.

CHAPTER THREE

ADVANCED MATERNAL AGE

Advanced maternal age (AMA) is defined as being 35 years or older on the estimated date of birth.

Risks associated with AMA:

- Aneuploidy
- Miscarriage
- Preterm birth
- Gestational diabetes
- Hypertensive disorders
- Placenta praevia
- Fetal growth restriction
- Stillbirth (SB)

Age	Risk of SB if giving birth for first time	Risk of SB if she has given birth before
under 35 years	3.72/1000	1.29/1000
35-39 years	6.41/1000	1.99/1000
40 and older	8.65/1000	3.29/1000

- risk of stillbirth increases with advancing gestational age
    - between 39 and 40 weeks, risk of SB is 1/1000 if she is < 35 years, compared to 1.4/1000 between ages 35-39 and 2/1,000 if the woman is 40 or older
    - the above risks are lower if she is healthy and does not have gestational diabetes (GDM) or hypertension. She is still at higher risk when compared to healthy women who are not AMA

- They have a higher rate of induction of labour and caesarean section

Antenatal care

- Recommend first trimester screen
- Offer non-invasive prenatal testing (NIPT)
- Monitor fetal growth and wellbeing

Birth plan

- Recommend induction of labour even though there are no trials with sufficient number to support this
  - in nulliparous women aged over 35
    - offer induction between 40^0-40^6 weeks
  - in nulliparous and multiparous women aged ≥ 40 years
    - offer induction at 39^0-39^6 weeks
- If they decline induction of labour, recommend twice weekly CTG
  - further recommend not to let the pregnancy go past 41^6 weeks

Recommended Reading

1. Reddy UM, Ko CW and Willinger M. Maternal age and the risk of stillbirth throughout pregnancy in the United States. Randomized Controlled Trial. *Am. J. Obstet. Gynecol.* 2006 Sep; 195(3): 764-70
2. Walker KF, Bugg GJ, Macpherson M et al. and the 35/39 Trial Group. Randomized Trial of Labor Induction in Women 35 Years of Age or Older. *N. Engl. J. Med.* 2016 Mar 3; 374(9): 813-22.
3. Fonseca MJ, Santos F, Afreixo V et al. Does induction of labor at term increase the risk of cesarean section in advanced maternal age? A systematic review and meta-analysis. *Eur. J. Obstet. Gynecol. Reprod. Biol.* 2020 Oct; 253: 213-219.
4. Dong Y, Wang L, Lu Y et al. Factors affecting mode of delivery in women of advanced maternal age. *Biosci. Trends.* 2021 Mar 15; 15(1): 61-63.

CHAPTER FOUR

AMNIOTIC FLUID EMBOLISM

The woman will develop sudden peri partum cardiopulmonary shock. Amniotic fluid embolism (AFE) is associated with high maternal and perinatal mortality.

Risk factors include:
Older age, precipitate labour, caesarean or instrumental vaginal birth, placental abnormalities (praevia, abruption, accreta) and preeclampsia/ eclampsia

Clinical features

- AFE develops during labour or soon after birth
    - there is sudden onset of cardiorespiratory arrest
    - there is hypotension with evidence of respiratory compromise (dyspnoea, cyanosis, or peripheral oxygen saturation < 90%)
    - the woman may develop coagulation abnormality with risk of bleeding
    - she may get convulsions

Exclude

- Anaphylaxis
- Septicaemia
- Pulmonary embolism
- Myocardial infarct
- Aortic dissection
- Tension pneumothorax

Management

- Make a diagnosis of AFE by excluding other causes of cardiopulmonary collapse
- Utilise a multidisciplinary team-based approach
- Initiate cardiopulmonary resuscitation (CPR)

- Control haemorrhage and reverse coagulopathy. Use tranexamic acid and activate massive transfusion protocol as she may need platelets, plasma, fibrinogen, rFactor VII and blood
- Consider delivery if the fetus is alive or if delivery might make maternal resuscitation easier

Recommended Reading

1. McDonnell, N., Knight, M., Peek, M. J. et al. Amniotic fluid embolism: an Australian-New Zealand population-based study. *BMC Pregnancy Childbirth* 15, 352 (2015).
2. Amniotic fluid embolism. Rare Disease Database. National organisation for rare disorders 2019.
3. Fitzpatrick KE, van den Akker T, Bloemenkamp KWM et al. Risk factors, management, and outcomes of amniotic fluid embolism: A multicountry, population-based cohort and nested case-control study. *PLoS Med.* 2019 Nov 12;16(11):e1002962.
4. Pacheco LD, Clark SL, Klassen M, Hankins GDV. Amniotic fluid embolism: principles of early clinical management. *Am. J. Obstet. Gynecol.* 2020 Jan; 222(1): 48-52.

CHAPTER FIVE

ANAEMIA IN PREGNANCY

Definition:
Hb < 110 in first and < 105 g/L in second trimester

- severe if < 70 g/L
- very severe if < 40 g/L

Physiological anaemia seen in the late second and early third trimesters is a dilution effect. Failure of this to occur may indicate inadequate placental function, and an increased risk of pre-eclampsia and stillbirth.

Useful classification

- **Normocytic, normochromic** – MCV, MCH and MCHC are all normal: this is seen with acute blood loss, early iron deficiency anaemia, physiological anaemia (dilutional drop in haemoglobin), haemolysis, and chronic inflammatory disease
- **Microcytic hypochromic** – MCV, MCH and MCHC may be low: this is seen with iron deficiency, thalassaemia and with some haemoglobinopathies
- **Macrocytic, normochromic** – MCV is elevated but MCH and MCHC are normal: this is seen with megaloblastic anaemia as a result of vitamin B12 or folate deficiency, liver disease, and hypothyroidism

Types of anaemias:

1. **Iron deficiency (90%)**

- There will be a fall in MCV first, followed by a fall in mean corpuscular haemoglobin (MCH) and finally a drop in haemoglobin (Hb)
- If Hb or MCV are low
    - request a review of blood film, haemoglobin electrophoresis and serum ferritin levels
        - low serum ferritin (< 15 μg/L) is the most useful indicator of iron deficiency

  - in women at high risk of anaemia (such as previous anaemia, multiple pregnancy, short interpregnancy interval and JWs), check serum ferritin early in the pregnancy

Management

- **Oral iron** - initially recommend Ferrogradumate C, Fefol or FGF
  - if Hb > 100 g/L and serum ferritin < 15 mcg/L, recommend one tablet daily and if there are side-effects this may be reduced to one tablet 2-3 times a week. Advise women to take iron tablets before meals
  - if Hg > 70 g/L, recommend one tablet twice daily and check Hb in 4 weeks
    - if Hb rises to > 15g/l advise to continue taking oral iron
    - if not consider iron infusion
  - if Hb < 70 g/L in early pregnancy or < 90 g/L in late pregnancy
    - consider iron infusion
- **Iron infusion** – consider iron infusion for anaemia in the third trimester or after birth especially in non-compliant women
  - intravenous Ferinject (iron CARBOXY maltose) – 1000 mg per dose over 30 min
    - some women may get skin pigmentation and delayed minor side effects (muscle cramps, arthralgias, fever, chills, headaches, and dizziness)
- **Blood transfusion** – reserve blood for women with severe anaemia at ≥ 36 weeks

2. Megaloblastic – Vitamin B_{12} and Folate deficiency

- Usually folate deficiency
  - except in strict vegans, true vitamin B_{12} deficiency is unlikely despite the increased requirements of pregnancy
  - suspect it if:
    - low haemoglobin is associated with high mean corpuscular volume (MCV) of > 100 fL
    - large hyper-segmented neutrophils are seen on the film
    - there is falling platelet count (< 100000 / L)
  - monitoring serum vitamin B_{12} and folate levels may help (there is marked post prandial and day to day variation in levels)

    - measuring red cell folate is a more reliable indicator of folate deficiency
- Other possible causes of megaloblastic anaemia are:
    - coeliac disease, Crohn's, or gastric banding
    - familial (family history of B12 deficiency)

Management
- In strict vegans, recommend prophylactically the intramuscular injection of 1,000 micrograms (mcg) of vitamin B_{12} every 3 months and a 5mg tablet of folic acid once a day
- Recommend 5mg folic acid once a day to women who are on antiepileptic treatment (Valproate and Phenytoin), Sulfasalazine, Azathioprine or to those who have a bowel malabsorption condition
- In all other women recommend intramuscular injection of 1,000mcg of vitamin B_{12} on alternate days for 2 weeks for vitamin B_{12} deficiency and 5mg of folic acid daily for folate deficiency

3. Haemoglobinopathies

Alpha thalassaemia (autosomal recessive) – seen more in South East Asia, India, and Africa
- They may have one defective gene (alpha thal^{+} trait), both defective genes from one parent (alpha thal^{0} trait) or one defective gene from each parent (homozygous alpha thal^{+} trait)
- They may have three defective genes, 2 from one parent and one from the other
    - there is risk of mild to moderate fetal anaemia
- They may have all four defective genes (homozygous alpha thalassaemia)
    - there is risk of fetal anaemia with heart failure and hydrops

Beta thalassaemia (autosomal recessive) – seen more in women from Mediterranean and Middle East countries, South East Asia, and China.
- If only one beta gene is defective (H trait or H minor), they may develop mild microcytic anaemia in pregnancy
    - if both beta genes are defective (H major), there is risk of fetal anaemia with heart failure and hydrops

Laboratory diagnosis
- There will be very low MCV (55-65fl) with a disproportionately high red cell count ($> 5.5 \times 10^{12}$ / L)
- Haemoglobin electrophoresis will confirm Hb A_2 level of $> 3.5\%$

- If there is coexistent iron deficiency, HbA_2 level may not be elevated until iron deficiency is corrected
- If both parents are carriers, recommend chorionic villus sampling to confirm fetal status
- Involve a genetic counsellor and a physician in management

Sickle cell anaemia (autosomal recessive) – seen mostly in women from East and West Africa

Homozygous (SS)

- These women will often have haemoglobin levels of 60-80g/L
- They may get frequent pain crises from thrombotic tissue infarcts
    - crises are usually precipitated by dehydration, exertion, infection or pain
- They are at increased risk of preeclampsia, placental abruption, fetal growth restriction (FGR), preterm labour and venous thromboembolism (VTE)
- Manage these women in consultation with a haematologist and an obstetric physician
    - recommend low dose Aspirin (150mg at night) from about 7 weeks gestation and 5mg folic acid daily
    - recommend prophylactic antibiotics throughout pregnancy
    - monitor haemoglobin levels 4 times weekly
    - recommend iron only if there is evidence of iron deficiency
    - blood transfusion may be required if Hb < 60g/l
- Plan delivery at around 38-40 weeks gestation
- This condition is associated with high perinatal and maternal mortality

Heterozygous (AS)

- These women are usually asymptomatic
- They have an increased risk of having a urinary tract infection (UTI)

Recommended Reading

1. Short MW and Domagalski JE, Iron Deficiency Anemia: Evaluation and Management. *American Family Physician* 2013; 87(2): 99-102.
2. Flores CJ, Yong A, Knights E et al. Maternity iron, anaemia and blood management in South Australia: a practice-based evidence for clinical practice improvement. *Vox Sang.* 2020 Jul 7. doi: 10.1111/vox.12969.

3. Feleke BE, Feleke TE. The Effect of Pregnancy in the Hemoglobin Concentration of Pregnant Women: A Longitudinal Study. *J. Pregnancy*. 2020 Jun 3; 2020: 2789536.
4. Lewkowitz AK, Gupta A, Simon L. et al. Intravenous compared with oral iron for the treatment of iron-deficiency anemia in pregnancy: a systematic review and meta-analysis. *J. Perinatol*. 2019 Apr; 39(4): 519-532.
5. Cantor AG, Bougatsos C, Dana T et al. Routine iron supplementation and screening for iron deficiency anemia in pregnancy: a systematic review for the U.S. Preventive Services Task Force. *Ann. Intern. Med.* 2015 Apr 21; 162(8): 566-76.

CHAPTER SIX

ANTENATAL CARE FOR NORMAL RISK WOMEN

- Provide information that is easily understandable and accessible and is consistent to all pregnant women
- Recommend folic acid supplement – 500mcg daily – to women intending to become pregnant or as soon as pregnancy is diagnosed up to 12 weeks of gestation to reduce the risk of neural tube defect
    - compulsory food fortification – 3 slices of bread (100g) contain an average of only 120 micrograms of folic acid

First hospital antenatal visit – Midwife/GP

- Ideally before 10-12 weeks
- Identify any risk factors, medical and social, and refer appropriately
- For women with high BMI, offer intensive healthy eating and physical activity advice as it may reduce excessive weight gain in pregnancy
- Iron supplementation – do not recommend routine iron supplementation to all pregnant women
- Vitamin D supplementation – recommend 10 micrograms of vitamin D per day to:
    - women who have limited exposure to sunlight
    - women who do not eat oily fish, eggs, meat, vitamin D-fortified margarine or vitamin D-fortified breakfast cereal
    - women with BMI > 30kg/m^2
- Recommend Aspirin 150mg at night and calcium 600mg twice daily if there is risk factor for pre-eclampsia
- Regarding smoking:
    - be proactive
    - discuss risks of smoking in pregnancy
    - discuss this at each antenatal visit
    - discuss benefits of quitting and offer any written resources
    - offer QUIT LINE referral

- Advise that alcohol should be avoided completely
    - if they continue to drink alcohol advise not to have more than one unit per day
- Recreational drugs – provide advice on cessation
- Exercise in pregnancy – advise that walks are good but to avoid contact sports
- Identify women who may need additional care:
    - if they are at risk of domestic violence
    - if they are at higher risk of post-natal depression (use Edinburgh Post-Natal Depression Score [EPDS])
- Antenatal classes – these improve women's experience of birth and parenting and women also generally view antenatal classes positively

Gestational age

- Confirm and agree on the expected date of confinement early in pregnancy
- Ultrasound is a more accurate predictor of gestational age than the use of the date of the last menstrual period (LMP)
    - use crown-rump length (CRL) up to 84mm or head circumference if CRL is > 84mm

Examination:

- Measure height and weight and calculate and record the BMI
- Blood pressure – do not rely on a single high reading – recheck after 5-10 minutes
    - hypertension is generally defined as two raised readings 6 hours apart
- Systemic examination – focus especially on the cardiovascular system

First trimester screen

- Combined first trimester screen between 11^0-13^6 weeks for Down's syndrome includes:
    - measurement of nuchal translucency and levels of beta-human chorionic gonadotrophin and pregnancy associated plasma protein-A (PAPP-A)
        - a low PAPP-A is a level of < 0.4 MoM
            - a low PAPP-A by itself is associated with mid trimester miscarriage, pre-eclampsia, fetal growth restriction, preterm birth and intrauterine fetal death

- Offer second trimester serum screening (triple or quadruple test) between 15 and 20 weeks if missed above
- Offer a non-invasive prenatal test (NIPT) – this test is now available and screens for many chromosomal defects
- Newer markers that may become more routine include placental growth factor (PIGF) and soluble fms-like tyrosine kinase 1 (sFlt-1) levels, amongst many others being investigated
- Screen for gestational diabetes (GDM): recommend an early oral glucose tolerance test (GTT) for women with the following risk factors for gestational diabetes:
    - body mass index above 30kg/m^2
    - advanced maternal age (age > 35)
    - previous history of macrosomia (baby weighing 4.5kg or above)
    - previous history of gestational diabetes
    - family history of diabetes (first-degree relative with diabetes)
    - ethnic group from countries with a high prevalence of diabetes:
        - India, Pakistan, Bangladesh, or Middle Eastern countries

Anomaly scan: 18 to 20 weeks

- Usually performed between 18^0-20^6 weeks to detect structural anomalies – this should include measurement of cervical length

20 weeks visit

- Review history to confirm risk status
- Review results of investigations and act appropriately if any are abnormal
- Check BMI – follow local obesity protocol
- Check anomaly scan results:
    - if the placenta was low-lying, recommend a repeat scan at 34 weeks
    - if nuchal fold was ≥ 6mm or if there were ≥ 2 "soft markers" for aneuploidy, refer the woman to a tertiary centre

24 weeks onwards

- Discuss any concerns
- Reemphasise healthy lifestyle issues
- Assess for risk factors for fetal growth restriction at each visit
    - use a local protocol for guidance on growth scans

- Check blood pressure
- Measure fundal height (FH) at each visit and plot it on an FH chart
    - encourage the woman to empty her bladder if she has not done so in the last 30 minutes
    - position the woman in a supine position with a slight lateral tilt
    - identify the top of the fundus by gentle palpation
    - hold tape with the cm marking hidden and measure from the uppermost border of the uterine fundus to the uppermost border of the symphysis pubis, without applying pressure over the fundus
    - turn over tape to read the measurement and record FH to the nearest cm
    - recommend a growth scan if:
        - there is a single abnormal reading more than 3cm below/above the expected value
        - two successive readings are below/above the expected level
        - there is an abnormal trend
- Start discussing fetal movements and enquire about fetal movements at each antenatal visit
    - advise they contact a health worker immediately if they have any concern regarding fetal movements
- Advise all women to go to sleep on their side as one strategy to reduce stillbirths
- If her blood group is Rhesus D-negative, offer partner testing to determine if there is any need for anti-D prophylaxis

28 weeks

- Enquire about fetal movements and give general advice regarding fetal movements
- Enquire about any vaginal bleeding
- Measure blood pressure (BP); if BP at any stage is 140mm or above systolic or 90mm or above diastolic, persisting after 2 readings 5-10 minutes apart – refer to the hypertension chapter for further care
- Measure and plot FH as above
- Check results of 26-28-week tests:
    - haemoglobin and OGTT (fasting blood glucose ≥ 5.1 or 2 hrs > 8.7 indicates diagnosis of GDM)
        - recommend iron supplementation if haemoglobin (Hb) is low

- Offer anti-D immunoglobulin to non-sensitized Rhesus-negative women
- Offer advice on sleeping positions

32 weeks

- Discuss fetal movements (FMs), sleep position and smoking if necessary
- Measure BP
- Measure and plot FH

34 weeks

- Discuss FMs, sleep position and smoking if necessary
- Discuss any concerns
- Measure BP
- Measure and plot FH
- Recommend second dose of anti-D immunoglobulin to Rhesus-negative women
- Recommend immunisation against whooping cough
- Confirm presentation

36 weeks

- As above
- If fetus is presenting as a breech, discuss external cephalic version (ECV)
- Check Hb
- Check on any need for a Group B Streptococcus (GBS) screen based on past pregnancies or current pregnancy
- Discuss again expectations of labour and options for pain during labour
- Discuss breast feeding

38 weeks

- Measure blood pressure
- Measure and plot FH
- Confirm fetus is presenting as cephalic

40+ weeks

- Measure blood pressure
- Measure and plot FH
- Offer membrane sweep
- Review any need for assessment of fetal wellbeing (very high BMI)
- Book for induction of labour (IOL) at 41^6 weeks

From 42 weeks

- If a woman continues to decline IOL for postdates, recommend alternate day CTG and at least one scan for umbilical artery doppler and amniotic fluid assessment

Recommended Reading

1. Antenatal care: Antenatal care for uncomplicated pregnancies. Clinical guideline Published: January 2017 nice.org.uk/guidance/cg62. UK.
2. Australian Health Ministers' Advisory Council 2012, Clinical Practice Guidelines: Antenatal Care – Module 1. Australian Government Department of Health and Ageing, Canberra. http://www.health.gov.au/antenatal.
3. Downe S, Finlayson K, Tunçalp Ö, Gülmezoglu AM. Provision and uptake of routine antenatal services: a qualitative evidence synthesis. *Cochrane Database Syst. Rev.* 2019 Jun 12; 6(6): CD012392. doi: 10.1002/14651858.CD012392.pub2
4. Peahl AF, Smith RD, Moniz MH. Prenatal care redesign: creating flexible maternity care models through virtual care. *Am. J. Obstet. Gynecol.* 2020 Sep; 223(3): 389.e1-389.
5. Abraham C. Rethinking the Traditional Prenatal Care Model. *Obstet. Gynecol.* 2020 May; 135(5): 1024-1026.

CHAPTER SEVEN

ANTEPARTUM HAEMORRHAGE

Antepartum haemorrhages occur in 2-5% of pregnancies.

Causes

- Placental abruption – 22%
- Placenta praevia – 31%
- Indeterminate/uncertain origin – 47%
- Incidental
- Vasa praevia

1. Placental Abruption

Placental abruption accounts for about 30% of cases of antepartum haemorrhage (APH). It is seen in 5% of placentae when clinically not suspected. 20-35% are concealed and 65-80% are revealed haemorrhages.

Predisposing factors include:

- Increasing age and parity
- Past history of placental abruption
- Smoking and recreational drug use
- Essential hypertension and pre-eclampsia
- Sudden decompression of the uterus (rupture of membranes with polyhydramnios)
- Severe fetal growth restriction (FGR)
- Injury – commonly physical injury or a motor vehicle accident
- It may occur in association with low lying placenta

Diagnosis

- Most commonly women will present with abdominal pain and vaginal bleeding
- There is often some tenderness over the abdomen
- There may be irregular uterine activity

- There may be features of hypovolaemic shock depending on the severity of bleeding
    - the uterus may feel woody, hard
    - the fetus may be distressed or even dead if there is major placental abruption
    - there may be evidence of disseminated intravascular coagulation (DIC)
- An ultrasound is often not helpful in making a diagnosis of placental abruption
- The Kleihauer-Betke test is also not recommended as a diagnostic test except for the assessment of feto-maternal haemorrhage in women who are Rhesus negative

Prevention

- Avoid the above predisposing factors
- Recommend low dose Aspirin at ≤ 16 weeks of gestation
    - its beneficial effect is seen if previous placental abruption was associated with fetal growth restriction

Management

- Light bleeding from the edge of a normally situated placenta is not uncommon and does not compromise the fetus or the mother – such cases only require reassurance

Mild placental abruption – expectant management

- Admit for observation over 24 hours – the majority will settle spontaneously
- Advise women to abstain from vaginal sexual intercourse or any strenuous activity for a few days
- Recommend a scan to exclude FGR
    - if normal and there are no risk factors for FGR or stillbirth, await spontaneous labour at term

Severe placental abruption

- Correct hypovolaemia
- Test for and treat any coagulation defect
    - if there is intrauterine fetal death, aim for vaginal birth if possible
    - if however, there is major blood loss with hypovolaemic shock, multi organ failure and or coagulopathy, waiting for

    vaginal delivery may be riskier and a caesarean section may be indicated
  - if the fetus is alive, recommend an immediate caesarean section
- Manage for prevention and treatment of postpartum haemorrhage – see the chapter on postpartum haemorrhage

Recommended reading

1. Young JS, White LM. Vaginal Bleeding in Late Pregnancy. *Emerg. Med. Clin. North Am.* 2019 May; 37(2): 251-264.
2. Downes KL, Grantz KL, Shenassa ED. Maternal, Labor, Delivery, and Perinatal Outcomes Associated with Placental Abruption: A Systematic Review. *Am. J. Perinatol.* 2017 Aug; 34(10): 935-957.
3. Qiu Y, Wu L, Xiao Y, Zhang X. Clinical analysis and classification of placental abruption. *J. Matern. Fetal Neonatal Med.* 2019 Oct 13: 1-5.
4. Atallah F, Goffman D. Improving Healthcare Responses to Obstetric Hemorrhage: Strategies to Mitigate Risk. *Risk Manag. Healthc. Policy*. 2020 Jan 21;13: 35-42.
5. Waters JH, Bonnet MP. When and how should I transfuse during obstetric hemorrhage? *Int. J. Obstet. Anesth.* 2021 May; 46: 102973.

CHAPTER EIGHT

ANTIPHOSPHOLIPID SYNDROME

Antibodies that may be detected include:

- Lupus anticoagulant (she will also have a prolonged APTT)
- Beta2 glycoprotein
- Anti-cardiolipin antibodies (significant if the level is > 40U/ml)
- Antiphophatidyl serine

Definition of antiphospholipid syndrome (APS)

- Presence of at least one of the above antibodies preconceptually or on at least 2 occasions 12 weeks apart with one or more of the following:
    - thromboembolism (deep vein thrombosis [DVT] or cerebrovascular accident most commonly, not superficial venous thrombosis)
    - $\geq$ 3 first trimester miscarriages
    - $\geq$ 1 fetal death with normal morphology occurring in the second or third trimester – fetal death is usually associated with FGR and oligohydramnios
    - $\geq$ 1 preterm birth < 34 weeks gestation associated with pre-eclampsia or placental insufficiency

Classification

- Primary APS – there is an absence of any other related disease
- Secondary APS – occurs with other autoimmune diseases such as systemic lupus erythematosus (SLE)

Management during pregnancy

- Multidisciplinary approach
- Recommend low dose of Aspirin (150mg at night) from pre pregnancy
- Recommend Clexane from 5-6 weeks gestation and continuing up to 6 weeks postpartum as these women are at a high risk of thromboembolism
- Exclude anti Ro and anti La antibodies

- Recommend routine first trimester screen and a 20 week morphology scan
- Encourage the wearing of TEDs stockings throughout pregnancy and up to 6 weeks postpartum
- Advise against the use of oestrogen containing contraceptive methods

Recommended Reading

1. Ghembaza A, Saadoun D. Management of Antiphospholipid Syndrome. *Biomedicines*. 2020 Nov 17; 8(11): E508. doi: 10.3390/biomedicines8110508
2. Devreese KMJ. How to Interpret Antiphospholipid Laboratory Tests. *Curr. Rheumatol. Rep.* 2020 Jun 19; 22(8): 38. doi: 10.1007/s11926-020-00916-5.
3. Espinosa G, Cervera R. Current treatment of antiphospholipid syndrome: lights and shadows. *Nat. Rev. Rheumatol.* 2015 Oct; 11(10): 586-96.

CHAPTER NINE

ASTHMA IN PREGNANCY

Effect of pregnancy on asthma

- Flare ups tend to occur in the late second trimester
- These often occur after a viral infection and in women with a high BMI

Effect of asthma on pregnancy

- There is increased risk of congenital malformation such as cleft lip with or without cleft palate
    - these are not related to any medication
- There is increased risk of developing GDM if on high doses of steroids for a long period
- The risk of pre-eclampsia, low birth weight, preterm birth and stillbirth is also higher

Management

- Advise the woman to stop smoking if she does
- Aim for good control before falling pregnant
- Advise on the importance of compliance with medication during pregnancy
- Assess asthma control at each antenatal visit (some suggest the use of spirometry at each visit)
    - in severe cases there may be a need for oral steroids – use the lowest dose required to obtain adequate control
    - use of low dose Aspirin in pregnancy may cause bronchospasm
    - all drugs commonly used to treat asthma are safe in pregnancy and during breast feeding
- Low vitamin D level during pregnancy is a risk factor for asthma exacerbations
- Advise women to get vaccinated against influenza and whooping cough according to guidelines
- Monitor fetal growth in women with frequent attacks

Intrapartum management

- Manage them as normal
    - in severe cases one may consider a planned induction of labour (IOL) during a stable phase of asthma
- Ensure they have adequate hydration and pain control
- In women who have been on Prednisolone > 5mg/day for > 2 weeks prior to labour, recommend intravenous injection of Hydrocortisone 50-100mg every 6-8 hours to prevent adrenal crisis (they can resume oral steroids soon after birth)
- Prostaglandin E2 and Misoprostol are bronchodilators and thus safe to be used if required
- Syntometrine is safe to be used for the prevention of postpartum haemorrhage
- Avoid Prostaglandin F2α as it may cause bronchospasm
- Recommend regional anaesthesia rather than general anaesthesia

Breast feeding

- Children of asthmatics have a higher risk of developing atopic diseases, including asthma
- Breast feeding is protective

Recommended Reading

1. Murphy VE, Jensen ME, Gibson PG. Asthma during Pregnancy: Exacerbations, Management, and Health Outcomes for Mother and Infant. *Semin. Respir. Crit. Care Med.* 2017 Apr; 38(2): 160-173.
2. McLaughlin K, Foureur M, Jensen ME, Murphy VE. Review and appraisal of guidelines for the management of asthma during pregnancy. *Women Birth*. 2018 Dec; 31(6): e349-e357.
3. Robijn AL, Murphy VE, Gibson PG. Recent developments in asthma in pregnancy. *Curr. Opin. Pulm. Med.* 2019 Jan; 25(1): 11-17.
4. Popa M, Peltecu G, Gica N et al. Asthma in Pregnancy. Review of Current Literature and Recommendations. *Maedica (Bucur)*. 2021 Mar; 16(1): 80-87.
5. Vieira AC, Pité H, Morais-Almeida M. Asthma and pregnancy in the 2020 decade: still a matter of concern. *J. Matern. Fetal Neonatal Med*. 2021 Apr 29: 1-7.

CHAPTER TEN

BACTERIAL VAGINOSIS

This is a common vaginal infection.

- In pregnancy vaginal flora change from a predominant lactobacillus to predominantly anaerobic organisms (Mycoplasma, Ureaplasma and Gardnerella Bacteroides)
- Vaginal pH becomes very alkaline in pregnancy

Clinical features

- Bacterial vaginosis (BV) infection is often asymptomatic but may cause smelly vaginal discharge or mild vaginal irritation
- In women with a previous history of preterm birth, late miscarriage or prelabour rupture of membranes, recommend screening for BV during the second and third trimesters even if they are asymptomatic

Risks

- With BV there is an increased risk of miscarriage, preterm prelabour rupture of membranes, preterm labour, chorioamnionitis and postpartum endometritis
- BV is associated with a 2-3-fold increased risk of acquiring STIs including Chlamydia, Gonorrhoea, Herpes Simplex type 2 and HIV infection

Diagnosis

- Women may complain of a smelly vaginal discharge
- Vaginal fluid pH is > 4.5
- Clue cells are seen on a gram stain

Treatment

- Metronidazole 400mg twice daily for 7 days or 2g stat
    - although frequently used, some suggest that in pregnancy this may increase risk of preterm birth
- Clindamycin 300mg twice daily for 5-7 days may be the preferred drug in pregnancy

- Recommend retesting 4-6 weeks after initial treatment

Recommended reading

1. Yudin MH and Money DM. Screening and Management of Bacterial Vaginosis in Pregnancy N 211; SOGC *Clin. Prac. Guideline* 2017; 39(8): 184-191.
2. Jayaram PM, Mohan MK, Konje J. Bacterial vaginosis in pregnancy - a storm in the cup of tea. *Eur. J. Obstet. Gynecol. Reprod. Biol.* 2020 Oct; 253: 220-224.
3. Redelinghuys MJ, Geldenhuys J, Jung H, Kock MM. Bacterial Vaginosis: Current Diagnostic Avenues and Future Opportunities. *Front Cell Infect. Microbiol.* 2020 Aug 11; 10: 354.
4. Sonthalia S, Aggarwal P, Das S. et al. Aerobic vaginitis - An underdiagnosed cause of vaginal discharge - Narrative review. *Int. J. STD AIDS*. 2020 Oct; 31(11): 1018-1027.

CHAPTER ELEVEN

BREECH PRESENTATION

Incidence of breech presentation is about 3-4% in labour at term.

Risk factors for breech presentation include:

- Nulliparity and grand multiparity
- Uterine abnormality – bicornuate or subseptate uterus and fibroids
- Contracted pelvis
- Previous breech presentation – risk of recurrence is about 10%
- Early gestational age
- Breech with extended legs
- Fetal abnormality especially of the central nervous system (CNS)
- Fetal growth restriction (FGR)
- Placenta praevia
- Multiple pregnancy
- Polyhydramnios and oligohydramnios
    - in most cases there is not an identifiable cause

Antenatal Management

- Recommend a formal scan in all cases to:
    - confirm the type of breech
    - look for the possible cause, fetal or maternal
    - exclude hyperextended neck and low-lying placenta
        - recommend a caesarean section if hyperextension of the fetal head is greater than 135 degrees because of the increased risk of spinal (cervical) cord damage during vaginal delivery
    - estimate fetal weight and liquor volume

External cephalic version (ECV)

- If there are no contraindications recommend ECV – this significantly reduces the frequency of breech presentation at term and of caesarean section

    - in nulliparous women, perform ECV at around 36 weeks gestation
    - in multiparous women, perform ECV at 37 weeks gestation
- Success rate is reported to be about 40-50% in women in their first pregnancy and 60-70% in multiparous women
- Success is more likely if there is
    - a good pocket of fluid below the presenting part
    - high parity
    - normal amniotic fluid volume
    - a flexed rather than frank breech
    - a lateral fetal spine
- The risk of reversion back to breech is about 5%

Contraindications to ECV include:
- Obvious cephalopelvic disproportion
- Confirmed FGR with fetal compromise
- Severe proteinuric hypertension with fetal compromise
- Severe lethal congenital malformation
- Placenta praevia or recent antepartum haemorrhage
- Another indication for caesarean section already present

Procedure
- Provide written information
- Obtain written informed consent
- Confirm fetal wellbeing – ensure cardiotocography (CTG) is normal
- Tocolytic agents improve the success rate:
    - one option is intravenous Salbutamol (500 micrograms given over 10-15 minutes very slowly – being guided by maternal tachycardia)
    - subcutaneous Terbutaline (250 - 500mcg) may also be used
- Use either talcum powder or gel on the abdomen – the use of gel has been reported to have a higher success rate than powder
- Gently manually dislodge the breech from the maternal pelvis and apply gentle pressure on the fetal head and breech to encourage a 'forward roll' or 'backward roll'
- Avoid persevering for too long
- Cease procedure if it's too uncomfortable or painful
- Administer 625 IU Anti-D immunoglobulin if Rh negative and they have not had the immunoglobulin in the last 2 weeks
- Ensure fetal wellbeing after ECV attempt, until CTG is normal

- As the risk of reversion back to breech is about 5%, encourage women to remain mobile and advise they empty their bladder frequently
- If ECV is initially unsuccessful, offer a second attempt or consider a second attempt under regional block

Complications of ECV include:

- Discomfort or pain
- Side effects from the use of a tocolytic agent
- Transient fetal bradycardia from cord compression
- Silent feto-maternal haemorrhage – risk is about 2%
- Rupture of membranes or onset of labour in about 5%
- Very rarely a prolonged bradycardia – if this occurs resort to immediate caesarean section
- Very rarely placental abruption – 1 in 1000

Vaginal breech delivery

- In selected cases and with the use of a strict protocol and presence of an experienced accoucheur, recent studies have shown that fetal/neonatal mortality or serious neonatal morbidity after vaginal birth is not significantly different from birth by a planned caesarean section
- Consider vaginal breech birth if women request it after adequate counselling and with informed consent
    - there is no evidence of benefit for routine use of pelvimetry
    - risks of vaginal birth include injury to abdominal viscera, fetal trauma (fractures) and difficulty with delivery of the head (thus the need for an experienced accoucheur).

Labour

- Await spontaneous onset of labour – induction of labour is not contraindicated
- Avoid early amniotomy
- Recommend continuous electronic fetal heart rate monitoring
- Ensure she is making adequate progress in labour (cervical dilatation and descent of presenting part) – any delay may indicate fetopelvic disproportion
- Fetal blood sampling from the buttocks during labour is not recommended
- Fetal scalp electrode may be applied to the buttock if external monitoring is unsatisfactory

- Epidural analgesia is useful but it is not a prerequisite
    - it relieves pain
    - it prevents involuntary pushing before full cervical dilatation
    - it provides immediate anaesthesia if a caesarean section or an obstetrical manoeuvre is required
- Augment labour only to initiate or strengthen weak contractions
    - do not use it for slow progress in the active phase of labour
- Discourage active pushing until the breech has descended to the pelvic floor
- Some women may request to birth on all fours, standing, or on a birth stool; these are safe positions to birth
- There is no need for a routine episiotomy but it is recommended if forceps are required to deliver the head
- With assisted vaginal breech birth, allow as much spontaneous delivery by uterine action and maternal effort as possible
    - intervene only to correct any deviation from the normal mechanism of spontaneous delivery
- Recommend immediate caesarean section in the presence of any significant fetal heart rate abnormality

Recommended Reading

1. Royal College of Obstetricians and Gynaecologist (RCOG). The management of breech presentation. London (UK). RCOG. December 2017.
2. Penn Z. Breech presentation. In: James D, Steer PJ, Weiner CP, Gonik B, Crowther C, Robson SC, editors. *High risk pregnancy management options*. Fourth ed. Philadelphia: Elsevier; 2011. p. 1101-1121.
3. Bin YS, Roberts CL, Ford JB, and Nicholl MC. Outcomes of breech birth by mode of delivery: a population linkage study. *Aust. N. Z. J. Obstet. Gynaecol.* 2016; 56: 453.
4. Goffinet F, Carayol M, Foidart JM, et al. PREMODA study group - Is planned vaginal delivery for breech presentation at term still an option? Results of an observational prospective survey in France and Belgium. *Am. J. Obstet. Gynecol.* 2006; 194: 1002.
5. Devold Pay AS, Johansen K, Staff AC, et al. Effects of external cephalic version for breech presentation at or near term in high-resource settings: A systematic review of randomized and non-randomized studies. *Eur. J. Midwifery.* 2020 Nov 20; 4: 44. doi: 10.1833.

6. Pulido Valente M, Carvalho Afonso M, Clode N. Is Vaginal Breech Delivery Still a Safe Option? *Rev. Bras. Ginecol.* Obstet. 2020 Nov; 42(11): 712-716.
7. Savchenko J, Lindqvist PG, Wendel SB. External cephalic version for breech presentation: The guideline landscape and a quest for an optimal approach. *Eur. J. Obstet. Gynecol. Reprod. Biol.* 2020 Dec; 255:197-202.
8. Toijonen A, Heinonen S, Gissler M, Macharey G. Risk factors for adverse outcomes in vaginal preterm breech labor. Arch Gynecol Obstet. 2021 Jan; 303(1): 93-101.
9. Martel-Santiago CR, Arencibia-Díaz RD, Romero-Requejo A et al. Delivery in breech presentation: Perinatal outcome and neurodevelopmental evaluation at 18 months of life. *Eur. J. Obstet. Gynecol. Reprod. Biol.* 2020 Dec; 255: 147-153.
10. Sánchez-Romero J, García-Soria V, Araico-Rodríguez F et al. External Cephalic Version: Is it an Effective and Safe Procedure? *J. Vis. Exp.* 2020 Jun 6; (160). doi: 10.3791/60636.

CHAPTER TWELVE

CAESAREAN SECTION

Timing of elective caesarean section (CS)

- Optimum time for repeat elective CS appears to be at 39-40 weeks of gestation, providing the lowest rate of an adverse neonatal outcome while minimizing the risk of spontaneous labour
- With previous classical incision there is no consensus regarding timing of CS
    - most would recommend CS at 37-38 weeks to reduce the possible risk of uterine rupture associated with onset of spontaneous labour

Preparation for CS

- Recommend a preoperative anaesthetic appointment particularly if there are anaesthetic issues of concern
- Check Hb if it hasn't been done in the last 4 weeks
- Send blood for group and hold for low risk cases
- Advise women to have preadmission shower using an antiseptic soap
    - this reduces risk of surgical site infection (SSI)
- Provide written information
    - advise women not to shave pubic hair but to clip if necessary
    - clipping can be performed on arrival in operating theatre
- Recommend use of prophylactic antibiotics
    - administer a single intravenous dose of Cefazolin 2g (3g if BMI > $30kg/m^2$)
        - if they are allergic to Penicillin, recommend Clindamycin (600mg)
    - recommend antibiotics to be given 15-60 minutes prior to skin incision
- Insert indwelling urinary catheter in the theatre, immediately pre-operatively, or in the ward prior to going to the theatre
    - recommend preoperative vaginal cleansing- soak a gauze swab in 10% povidone-iodine solution and insert into the distal vagina. The sponge holder and gauze should then be

rotated 360 degrees for 10 seconds from the vaginal vault to introitus - to reduce risk of endometritis particularly in women with ruptured membranes

- Preoperative skin cleansing
  - recommend using alcoholic Chlorhexidine rather than alcoholic Povidone-iodine
    - allow skin to dry spontaneously (usually 2 minutes) before draping
- There is no benefit to the use of separate knives for skin and deeper tissues

Caesarean section technique

- Skin incision
  - perform a suprapubic incision (in morbidly obese women consider a supraumbilical transverse incision)
  - using a scalpel rather than electrocautery is recommended
- Subcutaneous tissue layer
  - blunt dissection (with fingers) rather than sharp dissection (with a knife) is recommended
    - it is associated with shorter operative times
    - there is less chance of injury to blood vessels
- Fascial layer
  - make a small transverse incision in the middle with the scalpel, and then extended laterally with scissors
    - extending bluntly by fingers may increase risk of injury to blood vessels and muscle fibres
- Peritoneum
  - use fingers for blunt entry into peritoneal cavity to minimize the risk of inadvertent injury to bowel or bladder
  - use assistant to then open the rest of the peritoneum by pulling up-down and not laterally as the latter may cause bladder injury if it is adherent to the peritoneum
- Alexis retractor
  - its use in women with BMI > 35 provides good access
- Bladder flap
  - there is no advantage to routinely creating a bladder flap as this may cause haematoma formation
    - recommend this only if a difficult delivery is anticipated or if there are extensive adhesions

- Uterine incision
    - perform a transverse incision along the lower uterine segment
    - first perform a wide smiley superficial incision with a knife along the lower segment to reduce risk of tears into the angles
    - then make a transverse incision in the midline to gain entry into the uterine cavity
    - enlarge this opening through blunt transverse extension or through a caudal-cephaloid extension which is associated with less extension and bleeding
    - if a larger incision is needed perform a "J" extension
    - an upper segment incision (classical) may be needed for:
        - very preterm breech birth
        - back down in transverse lie
        - fibroids in lower uterine segment
        - dense bladder adhesions
- Delivery of head
    - in uncomplicated CS
        - gently flex the head with pressure over the occiput to deliver the head
        - can use forceps if needed
    - if head is deeply impacted (after prolonged second stage or failed instrumental delivery or second stage labour)
        - use of a fetal pillow
            - use this as a first choice especially with second stage CS
        - if the head is deeply impacted, deliver the anterior shoulder and arm first, then rotate the fetus and deliver the posterior shoulder and arm, followed by the fetal trunk, breech, lower limbs and finally the head
    - if the head is floating above the lower segment
        - use a vacuum or forceps
    - if a transverse lie
        - and the fetus is in the dorsosuperior (back up) position, deliver as a footling breech through a low transverse incision
        - and the fetus is in dorsoinferior (or back down) position you may need to perform a vertical incision in the uterus

- Cord clamping
  - delayed cord clamping is recommended as it results in higher neonatal haemoglobin levels for both preterm and term infants
- Cord gases
  - send arterial and venous cord blood gases for all emergency CSs and in other selected cases where there may be concern over fetal oxygenation
- Delivery of placenta
  - with placenta praevia
    - avoid disrupting the placenta when entering the uterus but if this is unavoidable, deliver the baby rapidly and clamp the umbilical cord promptly
  - perform controlled cord traction (CCT) or allow spontaneous expulsion (gentle traction on the cord after oxytocin injection)
    - avoid manual extraction
  - explore the uterine cavity to remove any remaining membranes or placental tissue using a dry sponge in one hand, using the other hand over the fundus to stabilize the uterus
- Prevention of postpartum haemorrhage (PPH)
  - use intravenous injections of Syntocinon (3 units slowly and repeat every 2-3 minutes if required)
  - other options include:
    - 100mcg Carbetocin (Duratocin) intravenously over 1 minute
    - 1g Tranexamic acid intravenously – evidence of its use to reduce haemorrhage is conflicting
  - massage the uterus after delivery of the placenta
  - recommend 30 Units Syntocinon in 500ml of Hartmann's solution over 4 hours
- Exteriorisation of uterus during closure
  - exteriorization may cause more nausea and more pain on the first postoperative day
- Uterine closure:
  - recommend a two-layer continuous closure
    - use a non-locking delayed absorbable suture
      - although in the short term there is no difference between one and two layer closures, a single layer closure may increase the risk of a uterine rupture in future pregnancy

                - a barbed wire suture may offer some advantage
    - during closure of the uterine incision recommend muscle to muscle closure and avoiding the endometrium
        - this policy may reduce risk of future morbid adherence of the placenta
- Routinely check ovaries and tubes
    - use a swab on a stick to mop paracolic gutters as it is less traumatic for the bowel compared to using a large abdominal sponge
- Peritoneal closure
    - visceral peritoneum – avoid closing this layer as this may be associated with haematoma formation and infection
    - parietal peritoneum
        - non closure is associated with greater adhesion formation
            - recommend closing the parietal peritoneum using an absorbable suture
- Rectus sheath closure
    - carefully check for any bleeding under the sheath prior to closing the rectus sheath
    - use a continuous non locking slow absorbing suture – 1/PDS or 1/Vicryl
- Subcutaneous tissue
    - subcutaneous closure is recommended if the layer is $\geq$ 2 cm; include the scarpa's fascia
        - this significantly reduces the risk of wound disruption and infection
- Skin
    - staples take less time than subcuticular sutures
        - their use doubles the risk of wound complications
        - women do not like staples
    - recommend continuous closure with 3/0 Monocryl
    - one can use Dermabond as a tissue adhesive to close the skin
- Wound dressing
    - current data do not show any benefit with routine use of negative pressure dressings
    - a systematic review showed reduction in SSI in women with high BMI

- Post-operative vaginal cleansing
  - after swabbing any blood in the vagina, end by cleansing the vagina with aqueous Povidone-iodine as this may further reduce the risk of endometritis

Postnatal care

- Offer NSAIDs (suppositories) postoperatively
- The anaesthetist may give spinal opiates and/or a patient controlled analgesia (PCA) for postoperative pain relief
- Offer lactational support if required
- Most women may have a light to normal diet as soon as they feel hungry or thirsty
  - there is no need to wait for or listen for bowel sounds
  - chewing gum accelerates return of normal bowel movements
- Remove the indwelling catheter (IDC) as soon as they are mobile but earlier than 12 hours from the last epidural top-up or spinal analgesia
- Check haemoglobin the next day ONLY in selected cases
- Debrief the woman and include options for future birth(s)
- Inform her General Practitioner

VTE prevention

- See relevant chapter on venous thromboembolism

Complications of CS
Short term

- Infection
  - endomyometritis, SSI (2-3%) – 40% occur after discharge from hospital
  - septic pelvic thrombophlebitis – ovarian vein thrombophlebitis (fever and abdominal pain develop within one week of surgery with thrombosis of the right ovarian vein) and deep septic pelvic thrombophlebitis
    - women present within a few days of surgery with unlocalized fever that persists despite antibiotics and negative scans
- Haemorrhage – 2 to 3% of women having a CS require a blood transfusion
- Urinary tract or bowel injury
  - this occurs in < 1% of cases (risk of cystotomy is higher for repeat elective caesarean sections and for CSs performed in the second stage)

- Ileus
    - rarely some women develop Ogilvie's syndrome (acute colonic pseudo obstruction)
- Venous thrombosis and pulmonary embolism
- Wound dehiscence
- Iatrogenic prematurity
- Birth trauma
- Transient tachypnoea of the newborn (TTN) and respiratory distress syndrome (RDS)
    - this is more after a planned elective CS
- Maternal mortality

Long Term

- Abnormal placentation
    - there is an increased risk of placenta praevia (1 in 200)
    - there is an increased risk of placenta accreta (risk increases with increasing numbers of prior CSs)
- Scar complications: ectopic pregnancy, numbness or pain, incisional endometriosis
- Uterine rupture in a subsequent pregnancy
    - inter-delivery interval of ≤ 24 months and single layer closure have been associated with an increased risk of uterine rupture
- Adhesions
    - may be asymptomatic or can cause significant morbidity and mortality as a result of bowel strangulation, obstruction and/or organ injury during repeat abdominal surgery

Recommended Reading

1. The CORONIS Collaborative Group. Caesarean section surgical techniques (CORONIS): a fractional, factorial, unmasked, randomised controlled trial. *Lancet* 2013; 382: 234–48.
2. The CAESAR study collaborative group. Caesarean section surgical techniques: a randomised factorial trial (CAESAR). BJOG 2010; 117: 1366–1376.
3. Dahlke JD, Mendez-Figueroa H, Rouse DJ, et al. Evidence based surgery for caesarean delivery: an updated systematic review. *Am. J. Obstet. Gynecol.* 2013; 209: 294-306.
4. Gillespie BM, Webster J, Ellwood D et al. Closed incision negative pressure wound therapy versus standard dressings in obese women

undergoing caesarean section: multicentre parallel group randomised controlled trial. *BMJ.* 2021 May 5; 373: n893. doi: 10.1136/bmj.n893.

5. Sentilhes L, Sénat MV, Le Lous M. et al. Tranexamic Acid for the Prevention of Blood Loss after Cesarean Delivery. *N. Engl. J. Med.* 2021 Apr 29; 384(17): 1623-1634.
6. Agarwal S, D'Souza R, Ryu M, Maxwell C Barbed vs conventional suture at cesarean delivery: A systematic review and meta-analysis. *Acta. Obstet. Gynecol. Scand.* 2021 Jun; 100(6): 1010-1018.
7. Carbone L, Saccone G, Conforti A. et al. Cesarean delivery: an evidence-based review of the technique. *Minerva. Obstet. Gynecol.* 2021 Feb; 73(1): 57-66.
8. Mireault D, Loubert C, Drolet P et al. Uterine Exteriorization Compared With In Situ Repair of Hysterotomy After Cesarean Delivery: A Randomized Controlled Trial. *Obstet. Gynecol.* 2020 May; 135(5): 1145-1151.

CHAPTER THIRTEEN

CARDIAC DISEASE IN PREGNANCY

Cardiac disease affects approximately 0.2% to 4% of pregnant women.

Cardiac diseases include

- Rheumatic heart disease
- Congenital heart disease
- Arrhythmias
- Ischemic heart disease
- Cardiomyopathy

Concerns specifically in cardiac cases include

- Pulmonary oedema
- Pulmonary hypertension
- Infective endocarditis
- Thromboembolism
- Peripartum cardiomyopathy
- Arrhythmias

New York Heart Association Classification

- Class I – no exertional dyspnoea – no limitation of physical activity
- Class II – dyspnoea on significant exertion – slight limitation of physical activity
- Class III – dyspnoea with mild exertion – marked limitation of physical activity
- Class IV – dyspnoea while resting

Heart conditions that require special care include

- Mitral stenosis
- Marfan's syndrome
- Pulmonary hypertension
- Complex congenital heart disease
- Women with mechanical valves

Management

Multidisciplinary team - Consult with anaesthetists, a cardiologist/obstetric physician

- The woman may need to consider not continuing with the pregnancy in some severe cases
    - generally, avoid pregnancy or continuation of pregnancy for women with:
        - pulmonary arterial hypertension, severe mitral stenosis, severe symptomatic aortic stenosis, severe aortic dilatation, vascular Ehlers Danlos and severe ventricular dysfunction

Antenatal

- As plasma volume increases in the third trimester, this is the time when risk of cardiac failure is higher
- If the mother has congenital heart disease
    - the fetus has an increased risk of having a congenital heart disease (3% versus 1% in the general population) with a 50% chance of having the same anomaly
    - apart from the normal morphology scan, arrange for a specialised fetal cardiac scan
- Recommend ECHO in the first and third trimesters as a minimum to detect any deterioration early
- Optimise cardiac medication as required
- Avoid anaemia
    - recommend oral iron supplementation
- Recommend anticoagulation
    - if prosthetic or mechanical valves are present
        - anticoagulate fully (ensure a PTT is twice normal)
            - use Clexane throughout the pregnancy
            - can also use a Clexane – Warfarin – Clexane regimen
    - recommend 150mg Aspirin daily at night in addition to above
- Treat any infection aggressively as it may predispose to cardiac failure
- Have a low threshold for thromboprophylaxis in pregnancy
- Monitor weight gain and recommend the avoidance of excess weight gain
- They have a higher risk of fetal growth restriction and preterm labour
    - monitor fetal growth
- Plan birth

    - recommend vaginal birth for most cases
    - wherever possible aim for spontaneous onset of labour
        - in some cases, a planned IOL may be required
- Discuss the need for antibiotic prophylaxis in labour

Labour and delivery

- Notify the physician, anaesthetist and obstetric consultants on call
- Use a Syntocinon infusion for induction or augmentation of labour or prostaglandin E2 if indicated
- Use a low volume Syntocinon infusion in women with a risk of fluid overload
- Ensure intravenous access
- Maintain a continuous midwifery presence
- Check recent haemoglobin, platelets, Chem 20 and APTT if anticoagulation medication is being used
- Advise her to adopt a lateral or upright position if on a bed
- Maternal monitoring in labour includes:
    - quarter to half hourly pulse, blood pressure, respiratory rate and pulse oximetry
    - hourly fluid balance to avoid fluid overload
    - continuous ECG for arrhythmias (telemetry)
    - continuous fetal heart rate monitoring for obstetric indication
- Analgesia
    - recommend an epidural – monitor blood pressure (hypotension is hazardous if they have a fixed cardiac output condition):
        - aortic stenosis
        - fixed mitral stenosis
        - hypertrophic cardiomyopathy
- Prophylactic antibiotics:
    - generally, do not recommend routine antibiotic prophylaxis for women undergoing an uncomplicated vaginal birth
    - intrapartum antibiotic prophylaxis is recommended with:
        - prosthetic heart valves
        - complex congenital heart disease
        - a past history of endocarditis
        - surgically constructed systemic-pulmonary shunts
            - recommend intravenous injection of 3g Ampicillin (2g Amoxycillin) 1.5mg/kg (over 30 minutes) and then 8 hourly for 24 hours after birth

        - for those who are allergic to Penicillin, use an intravenous injection of 1g of Vancomycin (over 60 minutes) and 80mg Gentamycin 8 hourly for 24 hours

- Manage the second stage as usual
- Avoid use of local anaesthetic with adrenaline
- Limit the number of vaginal examinations
- Avoid stirrups without discussion between the obstetrician, anaesthetist and cardiologist / physician
- Call the medical team if pulse rate > 130 or < 40bpm, or if respiratory rate > 24 or < 5rpm
- Avoid a prolonged second stage especially if there is a major risk of cardiac failure or if she has hypertension
    - in some cases, assist the second stage to avoid maternal effort; it is safe to use either a vacuum or forceps
- At the third stage
    - continue close monitoring up to the first 24 hours
    - recommend active management to prevent postpartum haemorrhage
        - avoid ergometrine as it can cause a sudden increase in cardiac return and cause decompensation
        - administer an intramuscular or intravenous injection of 5 units of Syntocinon
- Review 6 weeks postpartum to discuss contraception

Recommended Reading

1. ACOG Practice Bulletin No. 212: Pregnancy and Heart Disease, Obstetrics & Gynecology: May 2019 - Volume 133 - Issue 5 - p e320-e356 doi: 10.1097/AOG.0000000000003243.
2. Cardiovascular Diseases during Pregnancy (Management of) Guidelines, ESC Clinical Practice Guidelines 2018.
3. de Marvao A, Alexander D, Bucciarelli-Ducci C, Price S. Heart disease in women: a narrative review. *Anaesthesia*. 2021 Apr; 76 Suppl 4: 118-130.
4. Hutt E, Desai MY. Management of valvular heart disease in the pregnant patient. *Expert Rev. Cardiovasc. Ther.* 2020 Aug; 18(8): 495-501.

5. Ramlakhan KP, Johnson MR, Roos-Hesselink JW. Pregnancy and cardiovascular disease. *Nat. Rev. Cardiol.* 2020 Nov; 17(11): 718-731.
6. Davis MB, Arany Z, McNamara DM et al. Peripartum Cardiomyopathy: JACC State-of-the-Art Review. *J. Am. Coll. Cardiol.* 2020 Jan 21; 75(2): 207-221.

CHAPTER FOURTEEN

CHICKEN POX IN PREGNANCY

Primary chicken pox infection complicates about 3 in 1000 pregnancies. More than 90% of the population is seropositive and thus immune to chickenpox.

- Advise women who have not been exposed to be vaccinated prior to falling pregnant
    - after being vaccinated, advise her to avoid pregnancy for 3 months

Clinical features

- The incubation period is 1-3 weeks; she is infectious from 48 hours before the onset of the rash and persists until all lesions have crusted (4-5 days)
- She may have fever, malaise and a pruritic rash that becomes maculopapular and then develops vesicles that crust
- The virus remains dormant in sensory nerve root ganglia

Primary infection in pregnancy

Maternal risks

- Pregnancy increases the risk of severe illness
    - she can get oral lesions, fever, pneumonia (5-10%), hepatitis and encephalitis
    - the disease is more severe if the woman is infected later in pregnancy

Fetal risks

- Risk of miscarriage is not increased if she is infected in the first trimester
- There is an increased risk of preterm labour with infections later in pregnancy

- Concerning fetal varicella syndrome, the risk is
    - 0.5% if infected < 12 weeks gestation
    - 1.5% if infected between 12 and 28 weeks
    - 0% if infected after 28 weeks gestation
        - skin scarring in dermatome distribution, limb hypoplasia, eye defects, microphthalmia, cataracts and neurological abnormalities (microcephaly and mental retardation)
        - refer to a Maternal Fetal Medicine (MFM) specialist 5 weeks after the infection for discussion on amniocentesis and a scan
        - amniocentesis has a good negative but poor positive predictive value
        - if indicated, avoid performing amniocentesis until crusts have dried up
        - even if varicella virus PCR is positive, > 50% of infected women will give birth to a normal baby
    - offer an ultrasound scan to detect fetal infection after a lag time of at least 5 weeks
    - an MRI may also be helpful

Management if mother has primary chickenpox in pregnancy

- Avoid contact with other pregnant women and neonates until crusts develop (about 5 days after the rash)
- Offer symptomatic treatment to avoid secondary bacterial infection
    - if there are complications (respiratory symptoms, haemorrhagic rash, bleeding, new pocks developing > 6 days later, persistent fever for > 6 days or neurological symptoms)
        - admit into hospital – even if she has no complications but is in a high risk group (smoker, has chronic lung disease, was on systemic steroids in the last 3 months or she is > 20 weeks pregnant)
        - offer supportive therapy
        - recommend intravenous doses of 10mg/kg Acyclovir 8 hourly
    - if there are no complications
        - monitor at home as long as she has none of the risk factors mentioned above
        - if ≤ 24 hrs since the onset of the rash
            - offer 800mg Acyclovir orally 5 times a day for 7 days

        - if > 24hrs since the onset of the rash
            - Acyclovir is of no benefit
- Varicella zoster immunoglobulin (VZIG) given to the mother may prevent fetal varicella syndrome

Neonatal management

- If maternal infection occurs 1-4 weeks before birth, there is a 50% risk of neonatal infection and 25% of these infants will develop a clinical varicella infection
    - if maternal infection occurs > 7 days before birth
        - there is no benefit from VZIG
        - there is no need to advise isolation
        - breast feeding is safe
    - if maternal infection is within 7 days of the onset of the rash or if the rash starts within 2 days postpartum, there is a high risk of severe chickenpox in the newborn:
        - recommend 200 IU VZIG intramuscularly to the neonate at birth or within 72 hours
        - there is no benefit from isolation
        - it is safe to breast feed; if there are vesicles near the nipple, express breast milk until vesicles have crusted
        - discharge from hospital as soon as possible if term
    - if maternal infection occurs 2-28 days after delivery
        - if gestation age was < 28 weeks or if birthweight was < 1000g, recommend VZIG preferably within 96 hours (though it can be given up to 10 days post-maternal rash)
            - some recommend this for babies born at term as well
        - discharge term infants from hospital as soon as possible
        - there is no need to isolate the infant from the mother
        - it is safe to breast feed
            - 50% may get chickenpox despite VZIG
- Evaluate neonate for varicella infection until 28 days from the onset of the maternal rash
    - consider Acyclovir if it's a neonatal infection
    - recommend a neonatal ophthalmic examination at birth and test for IgM at birth and at 7 months

Neonatal contact

- If the newborn comes into contact with chickenpox
    - no action is required if the mother is IgG positive
    - offer VZIG if the mother is nonimmune

Health worker contact

- If they are nonimmune, recommend chickenpox vaccination

Management if the mother has contact with shingles

- Herpes zoster (shingles) is infectious if
    - it is disseminated
    - it is in an exposed area such as the eyes or thoraco-lumber region
        - if it is not in an exposed area, risk of transmission is very low
    - the person is immunocompromised (high viral shedding)

Management if the mother has contact with chickenpox

- If the woman has definitely had chickenpox or shingles in the past
    - no action is required (no need for IgG confirmation)
- If they're unsure whether or not they've had chickenpox or shingles, recommend testing for IgG
    - if immune, reassure her and no action is required
- If nonimmune or not able to get serology within 96 hours:
    - if exposure within ≤ 96 hours
        - recommend VZIG without waiting
        - advise they see a doctor if a rash develops
    - if exposure > 96 hours
        - VZIG is of no benefit
        - consider oral Acyclovir if in a high risk group as above
        - manage her as being potentially infectious for up to 28 days (21 days if not given VZIG)
        - if she is admitted to hospital for any reason, put her under airborne precautions in a single isolation room
    - a dose of VZIG is 125 U/10kg up to a maximum of 625 Units
    - vaccinate nonimmune women postpartum
- It is safe to breast feed

Recommended Reading

1. Shrim A, Koren G, Yudin MH, et al. Maternal Fetal Medicine Committee. Management of varicella infection (chickenpox) in pregnancy. *Journal of Obstetrics and Gynaecology Canada* 2012; 34: 287–92.
2. Lamont RF, Sobel JD, Carrington D et al. Varicella–zoster virus (chickenpox) infection in pregnancy. *BJOG*; 2011; 118: 1155–62.
3. Palasanthiran P, Starr M, Jones C, editors. Management of perinatal infections. Sydney: Australasian Society for Infectious Diseases (ASID); 2014.
4. Institute of Obstetricians and Gynaecologists, Royal College of Physicians of Ireland and the Clinical Strategy and Programmes Division, Health Service Executive. Clinical practice guideline, Chickenpox in pregnancy. Version 1.0 Publication date: Nov 2015 Guideline No: 19.

CHAPTER FIFTEEN

CORD PROLAPSE

Cord presentation is the presence of the cord in front of the presenting part whilst the membranes are intact.

Cord prolapse is the protrusion of the umbilical cord alongside (occult) or in front (overt) of the presenting part.

Maternal and fetal risk factors

- Rupture of membranes (spontaneous or during amniotomy) with high presenting part (all causes of high head)
- Malpresentation, especially a footling breech or transverse lie
- Multiparity – membranes rupture before contractions with head still high
- Multiple pregnancy, especially with second twin
- Preterm labour – relatively more liquor volume
- Polyhydramnios from any cause
- Fetal anomaly, especially anencephaly
- Cervical ripening with transcervical balloon catheters

Diagnosis

- If cord presentation is found on an ultrasound scan there is an increased risk of cord prolapse
    - the majority of such cord presentations are however not followed by cord prolapse
- Usually, it is diagnosed during a vaginal examination
    - the cord is palpable or visible at the introitus
    - with occult cord prolapse, there may be variable decelerations or fetal bradycardia
- Suspect a cord prolapse when there is sudden prolonged fetal bradycardia or a sudden change to persistent variable decelerations, especially if it follows soon after the rupture of membranes

Prevention

- Identify women at risk
- Perform speculum examination in at risk women immediately after the rupture of membranes
- With a transverse, oblique or unstable lie, consider admitting the woman into hospital after 37 weeks
    - if she is remaining at home, advise her to attend hospital immediately when her membranes rupture
- Avoid amniotomy with a high head, or if this is necessary, perform a controlled release of liquor with fundal pressure after informing the theatre
    - recommend using a small gauge needle or fetal scalp electrode to perform an amniotomy in such cases

Management

- Treat it as an obstetric emergency
- If on a Syntocinon infusion, cease the infusion
- Mode of birth will depend on whether the fetus is alive or not, on the gestational age, and on the stage of labour
    - if the fetus is not alive (confirmed by scan), aim for a vaginal birth
    - if gestational age is pre viable, aim for a vaginal birth
    - if she is in the second stage of labour and the presenting part is at or below the spine it may be possible to perform a quick spontaneous or assisted vaginal birth, especially in a multiparous woman
    - recommend a caesarean section in most cases
- While preparing for emergency caesarean section
    - position her in a steep Trendelenburg or in the knee-chest position to relieve compression of the cord
    - keep the vaginal hand in and use it to lift the presenting part up off the cord until the birth of the baby
    - avoid handling the cord to prevent a vasospasm
    - if she is not having strong contractions or if there might be some delay in performing a CS, rapidly fill the bladder with 500ml of normal saline while keeping her in the knee chest position
        - clamp the catheter and connect it to a urinary drainage bag
        - release the clamp to empty the bladder immediately prior to surgery

  - recommend 250mcg subcutaneous Terbutaline if she is in labour
- Obtain arterial and venous cord blood gases immediately after birth

Recommended Reading

1. Bord I, Gemer O, Anteby EY, Shenhav S. The value of bladder filling in addition to manual elevation of presenting fetal part in cases of cord prolapse. *Arch. Gynecol. Obstet.* 2011; 283: 989–91.
2. Sayed Ahmed WA and MA Hamdy. Optimal management of umbilical cord prolapse. *Int. J. Women's Health*. 2018; 10: 459–465.
3. Umbilical Cord Prolapse Green-top Guideline No. 50 RCOG 2014.
4. Pagan M, Eads L, Sward L et al. Umbilical Cord Prolapse: A Review of the Literature. *Obstet. Gynecol. Surv.* 2020 Aug; 75(8): 510-518.
5. Ahmed S, Hamdy MA Optimal management of umbilical cord prolapse. *Int. J. Women's Health.* 2018 Aug 21; 10: 459-465.

CHAPTER SIXTEEN

CYTOMEGALOVIRUS INFECTION

Incidence of cytomegalovirus infection is about 6/1000 pregnancies. The majority of the infections are asymptomatic – 50-60% of adults have been infected during childhood.

- The virus remains dormant for life
- Reactivation occurs in about 2% of women in pregnancy

Transmission is via contact with a person excreting the virus in the respiratory system, saliva, urine or bodily fluids.

- It can also be transmitted sexually, trans-placentally and via breast milk

Primary infection

- At risk women include those who have frequent prolonged contact with young children, day care workers and parents with a child in day care

Clinical feature

- The majority of maternal infections are asymptomatic
- The woman may have mild flu-like illness, rashes or gastrointestinal symptoms
- She may have lymphocytosis and mildly abnormal liver function tests

Diagnosis

- Serology
    - if IgG and IgM are negative, there is no infection
        - recommend retesting in 2-4 weeks if susceptible
    - if IgG is positive and IgM is negative, it indicates past exposure
    - if IgG is negative or if IgM is positive
        - recommend retesting in 2 weeks for seroconversion or a significant rise in IgG level (IgM antibodies can persist for 2-3 years)

            - if there is no change in IgG, it may be due to a possible recent infection
    - if IgG and IgM are positive, it could mean reinfection – this is associated with a rise in IgG antibody titre
        - recommend CMV specific IgG avidity – low avidity indicates a recent primary infection and high avidity indicates a past infection
- Amniocentesis for PCR and viral culture
    - is performed 6 weeks or more after primary maternal infection but not before 21 weeks gestation (low sensitivity)
    - and should be repeated if tests done prior to 21 weeks of gestation are negative (> 80% sensitive after 20 weeks)
- Ultrasound to detect fetal infection
    - features associated with symptomatic congenital CMV infection include microcephaly, hydrocephalus (ventricular dilation), fetal growth restriction, ascites, intracranial calcification, pleural or pericardial effusions, oligo or polyhydramnios, hydrops fetalis and hyperechogenic bowel
- Send placenta for histology – CMV inclusion antibodies will be seen in 10% of cases
    - this is associated with poor prognosis for the infant

Congenital CMV infection

- Risk of feto-maternal transmission is about 30% with primary infection
    - 85-90% of newborns are asymptomatic at birth with detection of the virus in amniotic fluid
        - 10% risk of sequalae
    - 10-15% are symptomatic
        - 50% risk of sequelae
- Features include fetal growth restriction, microcephaly, intracerebral calcification, hepatosplenomegaly and stillbirth
- At birth the newborn may develop petechiae, jaundice, chorioretinitis, thrombocytopenia and anaemia
    - 20% to 30% of them will die, mostly of disseminated intravascular coagulation, hepatic dysfunction or bacterial superinfection
    - 10% will develop symptoms in childhood – 85-90% of these will develop features during and up to the first few years of life

Non-primary CMV infection (reactivation or reinfection)

- IgG avidity assay can help to diagnose reactivation – virus-specific IgG of a low avidity is produced during the first months after the onset of infection
    - an avidity index > 60% is highly suggestive of past or secondary infection, while an avidity index of < 30% is highly suggestive of a recent primary infection (duration < 3 months)
- Risk of transmission of CMV to the newborn is about 1%
    - less than 1% of these will be symptomatic
    - a small percentage will later develop hearing loss and chorioretinitis
    - generally, if hearing is normal at one year of age, there is unlikely to be intellectual impairment

Management

- Counsel her regarding continuation or otherwise of pregnancy
- Have a paediatrician present at the birth
- Investigations in the newborn include:
    - serology for CMV and viral detection by PCR within the first few weeks
    - PCR and/or viral culture of urine and nasopharyngeal aspirate
    - an ophthalmology examination
    - a cranial ultrasound
    - a CT scan of the brain
    - a cranial MRI
- Follow-up all infants for at least the first 2 years

Prevention of fetal infection

- Current data do not support a role for CMV immunoglobulin in preventing in utero transmission of CMV
- Once fetal infection is diagnosed by amniocentesis, consider the use of specific hyperimmune globulin

Breastfeeding

- Benefits of breast-feeding (with primary or reactivation) outweigh the minimal risk of acquiring CMV through breast milk

Recommended Reading

1. Yankowitz J and Pastorek II Maternal and fetal viral infections. In: *High Risk Pregnancy* Eds. James DK, Steer PJ, Weiner CP and Gonik B. WB Saunders. 5th Edition 2016, pp. 534-38.
2. Palasanthiran P, Starr M, Jones C, editors. *Management of perinatal infections*. Sydney: Australasian Society for Infectious Diseases (ASID); 2014.
3. SOGC Clinical Practice Guideline. Cytomegalovirus Infection in Pregnancy. No. 240, April 2010. *J. Obstet. Gynaecol.Can.* 2010; 32(4): 348–354.

CHAPTER SEVENTEEN

DECREASED FETAL MOVEMENTS

- Many define normal fetal movements (FMs) as 10 movements in 2 hours at a time when the fetus is usually active
- 99% of women will feel 10 movements in 60 minutes
- FMs do not decrease but continue to term
- During fetal sleep cycles there are reduced FMs
    - these cycles last 20-40 min and almost never more than 90 minutes
    - perception of FMs can be affected by
        - high BMI
        - anterior placenta
        - smoking
        - alcohol and substance abuse
        - being busy and focusing on other matters, especially at work
- There is no clear definition of decreased fetal movements (DFMs)
    - if a woman has any concern about FMs, this should be taken seriously
- Women who have a stillbirth have often had varying periods of DFM prior to confirmation of fetal death
- DFM is associated with oligohydramnios, preterm birth, congenital malformations, chromosomal abnormalities, feto-maternal haemorrhage, abnormal neurodevelopment issues, placental insufficiency, and stillbirths
    - about 15% of women who report DFM have a growth restricted fetus

Management of women regarding fetal movements

- Enquire and document presence of normal FMs at every antenatal visit in the third trimester
- Advise women that if they have any concern about FM then they should contact the hospital immediately and not wait until the next day

- Widescale awareness of FM combined with guidelines on management of DFM has been shown to reduce stillbirth rate
- At any presentation with concern about FM:
    - assess history and progress to date in current pregnancy for risk factors associated with increased risk of stillbirth (poor past obstetric history, smoking, high BMI, advanced maternal age [AMA], hypertension, diabetes, small for gestational age fetus etc.)
    - perform clinical examination as usual, including measurement of blood pressure and fundal height (FH)
    - listen for FH to exclude fetal death
    - manage as per the flow chart shown below

Recommended Reading

1. Daly LM, Gardener G, Bowring V et al. Care of pregnant women with decreased fetal movements: Update of a clinical practice guideline for Australia and New Zealand. *Aust. N. Z. J. Obstet. Gynaecol.* 2018 Aug; 58(4): 463-468.
2. Akselsson A, Lindgren H, Georgsson S et al. Daily structured approach to awareness of fetal movements and pregnancy outcome - a prospective study. *Sex. Reprod. Healthc.* 2019 Jun; 20: 32-37.
3. Rådestad I, Doveson S, Lindgren H et al. Midwives' experiences of using the Mindfetalness method when talking with pregnant women about fetal movements. *Women Birth.* 2020 Oct 23: S1871-5192(20)30364-4.
4. Akselsson A, Lindgren H, Georgsson S et al. Mindfetalness to increase women's awareness of fetal movements and pregnancy outcomes: a cluster-randomised controlled trial including 39 865 women. *BJOG*. 2020 Jun; 127(7): 829-837.
5. Bellussi F, Po' G, Livi A et al. Fetal Movement Counting and Perinatal Mortality: A Systematic Review and Meta-analysis. *Obstet. Gynecol.* 2020 Feb; 135(2): 453-462.
6. Heazell AEP, Budd J, Li M, et al. Alterations in maternally perceived fetal movement and their association with late stillbirth: findings from the Midlands and North of England stillbirth case-control study. *BMJ Open*. 2018 Jul 6; 8(7): e020031. doi: 10.1136/bmjopen-2017-020031.
7. Linde A, Georgsson S, Pettersson K et al. Fetal movement in late pregnancy - a content analysis of women's experiences of how their unborn baby moved less or differently. *BMC Pregnancy Childbirth.* 2016 Jun 1;16(1):127. doi: 10.1186/s12884-016-0922-z. PMID: 27245990.

Decreased Fetal Movement Guidelines (DFM) – First Presentation

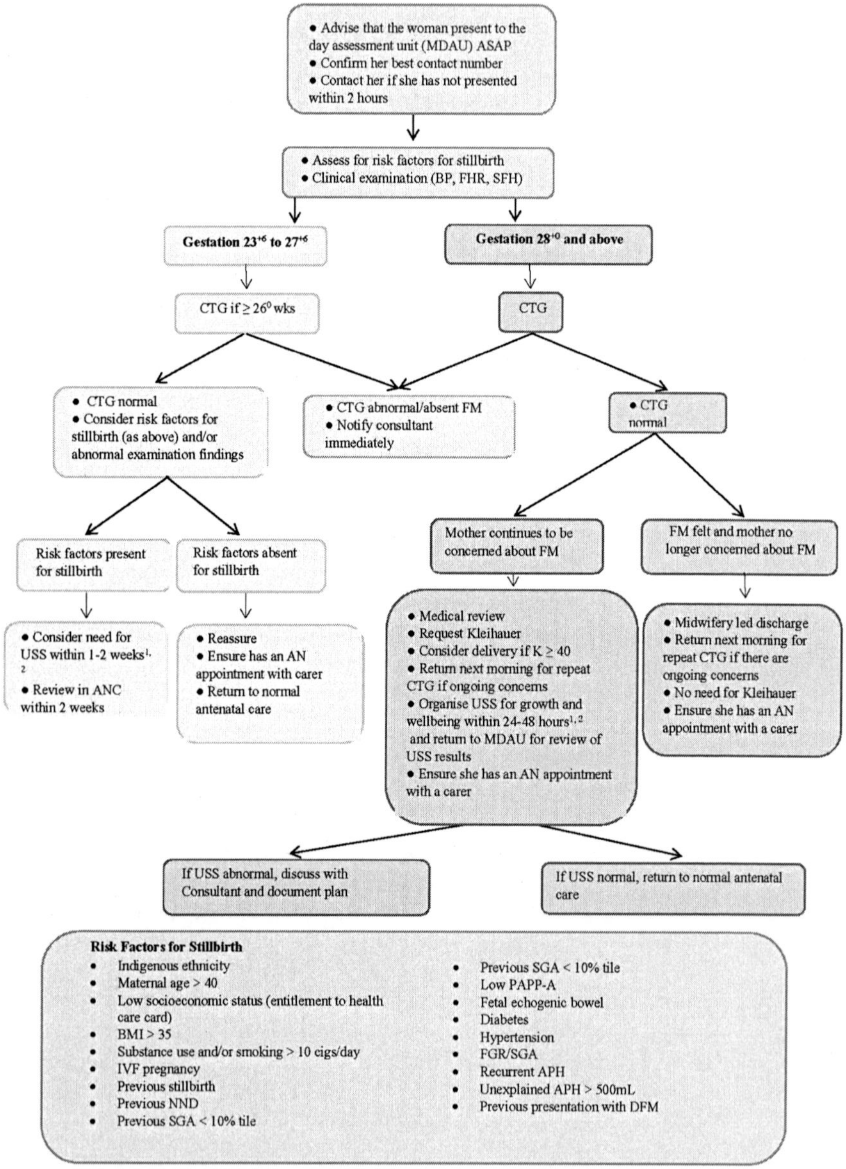

Decreased Fetal Movement Guidelines (DFM) – Second or Subsequent Presentation

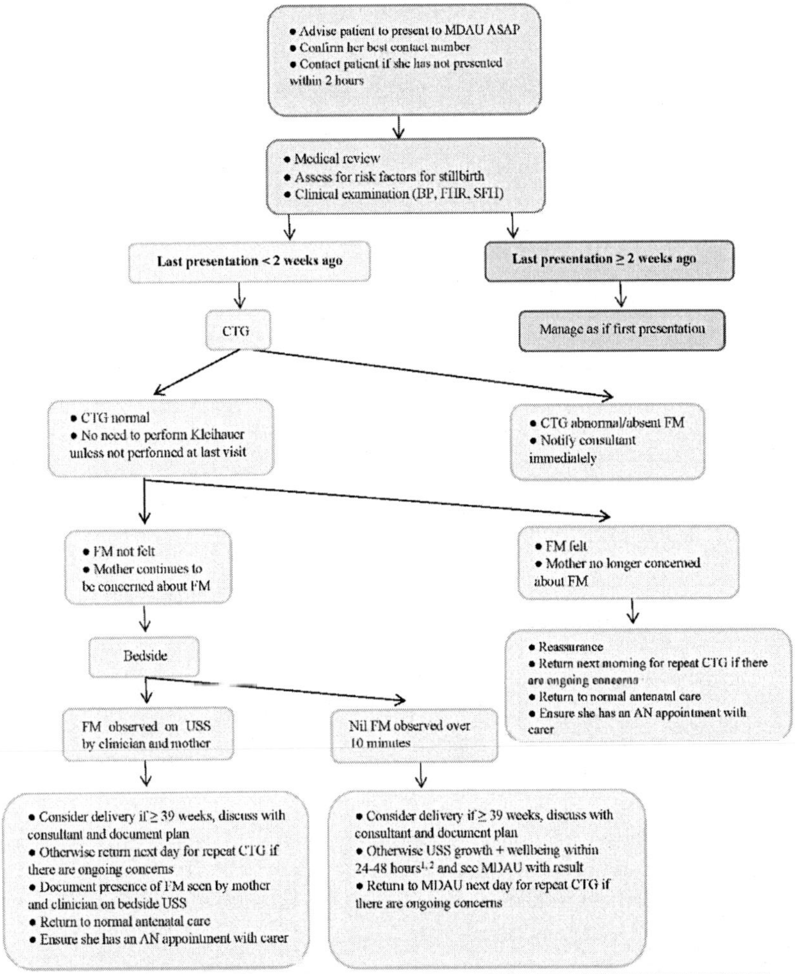

Risk Factors for Stillbirth

- Indigenous ethnicity
- Maternal age > 40
- Low socioeconomic status (entitlement to health care card)
- BMI > 35
- Substance use and/or smoking > 10 cigs/day
- IVF pregnancy
- Previous stillbirth
- Previous NND
- Previous SGA < 10% tile
- Previous SGA < 10% tile
- Low PAPP-A
- Fetal echogenic bowel
- Diabetes
- Hypertension
- FGR/SGA
- Recurrent APH
- Unexplained APH > 500mL
- Previous presentation with DFM

CHAPTER EIGHTEEN

DIABETES IN PREGNANCY

Pre-existing diabetes

Effect of pregnancy on diabetes

- Increasing doses of Insulin are required as pregnancy advances, especially around 28-32 weeks
- The woman may get hypoglycaemia, possibly from over control
- They may get ketoacidosis, often associated with infection, hyperemesis or use of corticosteroids

Effect of diabetes on pregnancy
Maternal:

- Macrovascular disease, coronary and cerebrovascular disease
- Microvascular disease may be diagnosed for the first time or if already present may worsen
    - o diabetic nephropathy (creatinine levels > 125umol/l)
    - o diabetic retinopathy (risk is doubled, especially with type 1 diabetes, and usually related to poor control as well as presence of hypertension and renal disease)
- Diabetic neuropathy
- Pre-eclampsia (3-4-fold increase, especially if they have chronic hypertension or renal disease)
    - o risk correlates closely with diabetes control in early pregnancy
- Infections – increased risk of UTI, respiratory infections, endometritis and SSIs
- Polyhydramnios: associated with poor control, it may lead to malpresentation, unstable lie and preterm labour
- Caesarean section

Fetal:

- Miscarriage (risk is 9-14% rate with preexisting diabetes and depends on degree of pre-pregnancy control)
    - good glycaemic control normalizes the miscarriage rate
- Congenital malformation
    - incidence is about 5% (double background), mainly of CNS (anencephaly, spina bifida), cardiac (VSD), sacral agenesis and renal anomalies
    - the rate is lower with good pre-conceptual control (5% if HbA1c levels are < 8% and up to 25% if > 8%)
        - aim to keep HbA1c level < 7%
- Macrosomia (birth weight > 4500 g or > 90th centile)
    - occurs in 15-45% of babies born to diabetic women
    - it is often an indication of poor control
    - obesity has a strong and independent effect on fetal macrosomia
    - fetal birth weight correlates best with second and third trimester fasting and postprandial blood sugar levels
    - macrosomia is associated with higher rates of neonatal morbidity (shoulder dystocia, severe hypoglycaemia and neonatal jaundice)
- Fetal growth restriction
    - it is more common in women with preexisting type 1 diabetes with vascular disease
- Polycythaemia – hyperglycaemia causes increased fetal erythropoietin production
- Hypoglycaemia
    - 15-25% of neonates delivered from women with diabetes in pregnancy develop hypoglycaemia in the first 12 hours after birth
    - it is less frequent when there has been tight glycaemic control during pregnancy and in labour
    - unrecognized hypoglycemia may cause seizures, coma and brain damage
- Hypocalcaemia
    - it occurs in up to 50% of infants secondary to functional hypoparathyroidism and it is dependent on the degree of diabetic control
- Hyperbilirubinaemia
    - it occurs in about 25% of infants due to prematurity, polycythaemia and trauma

- Respiratory distress syndrome, due to delayed lung maturation
- Sudden unexplained intrauterine fetal death – no test will predict this
- Increased perinatal mortality – especially with poor control and vascular disease

Management

Pre-pregnancy

- Use allied health for diet control, weight control and physical exercise
- Aim for strict pre-pregnancy control
    - fasting 4.0-5.9mmol/l
    - 1 hour postprandial < 7.8mmol/l
    - 2 hours postprandial < 6.8mmol/l
- Aim to maintain glycosylated haemoglobin < 7%
- Assess cardiovascular, renal and ophthalmologic status
- Advise on peri conceptual folic acid supplementation

Antenatal care

- See as early as possible, ideally by 10 weeks
- Advise on low dose of Aspirin, 150mg daily at night, and calcium 600mg twice daily
- Liaise with the physician, dietician and diabetic educator to get good control
- Recommend strict control especially during the first few weeks of pregnancy to reduce fetal congenital malformation
- Recommend a first trimester screen and /or NIPT
- Assess renal and liver function
- Assess thyroid function
- Monitor for any evidence of pre-eclampsia
- Recommend an ophthalmology assessment for type 1 diabetic women at booking and again in the early third trimester (repeat in 4-6 weeks if initially abnormal)
- Diabetic control – aim for:
    - fasting levels of < 5.1mmol/l
    - 2 hours post prandial levels to be < 6.7mmol/l
        - postprandial control predicts birthweight and neonatal hypoglycaemia better than pre-prandial control
    - monitor HbA1c monthly in early pregnancy and in those whose compliance may be poor (aim for levels <7%)
- Recommend an anomaly scan at 18-20 weeks
- Request a tertiary scan at 24 weeks

    - preferably request an ECHO at 22 weeks for type 1 and for type 2 if glycosylated haemoglobin is markedly elevated (> 10%), looking for cardiac abnormality
- Fetal growth and wellbeing
    - if on Insulin, recommend ultrasound scans for growth at 28-30 weeks and at 34-36 weeks
- See every 2-4 weeks depending on control up to 28 weeks, once or twice a fortnight until 36 weeks and weekly or more often thereafter if they require steroid loading, admit and monitor sugar and potassium closely, and use an insulin infusion
- Monitor for hypoglycaemia (educate on symptoms and what to do [sweets, sugary drinks, etc.])

Medication for diabetic control:

- Oral hypoglycaemics:
    - recommend Metformin (if not diet controlled), 500mg one to three times a day, depending on the glucose profile
        - it provides good blood sugar control and has similar outcomes in terms of a large for gestational age fetus (LGA), birth weights and neonatal complications
        - < 10% of women will require an addition of insulin to achieve glucose control

- Insulin is usually a combination of a short and intermediate type:
    - recommend two thirds at breakfast and one-third at bedtime (for the evening regime could be short acting at dinner time and intermediate at bedtime to prevent hypoglycaemia in the early morning) – a suggested regime could be:
        - if elevated fasting, only use a single dose of intermediate acting at bedtime (peak effect is in 4-12 hrs and lasts up to 24 hours)
        - if postprandial sugars are elevated, use rapid acting at mealtimes (starts acting within half an hour, peaks at 2-3 hours and lasts up to 4-5 hours)
        - if all are abnormal use rapid acting at mealtimes and intermediate acting at bedtime or a combination twice daily

Timing of delivery

- Type 1 and 2 uncomplicated diabetes
  - Recommend delivery at 38^0-38^6 weeks
    - in some cases, with poor control delivery may be indicated earlier
- If the woman is diet-controlled type 2 and there is no evidence of macrosomia
  - await spontaneous labour and offer IOL at 41^0-41^6 weeks as for post dates
- If there is evidence of macrosomia:
  - if estimated fetal weight (EFW) is > 3500g at 36 weeks or if
  - EFW is > 3700g at 37 weeks or if
  - EFW is > 3900g at 38 weeks
    - recommend induction of labour at 38^0-38^6 weeks
    - some data suggest avoiding induction of labour solely for isolated fetal macrosomia

Mode of delivery

- If EFW on scan is > 4500g recommend an elective caesarean section

Management in labour

- Inform the neonatal team
- Insulin infusion is not required for type 2 but is recommended for all type 1 diabetics
  - use a sliding scale, 2-6U/hr to maintain glucose level at 4-7mmol/l
- Recommend continuous fetal heart rate monitoring
- Anticipate shoulder dystocia

Postpartum

- It is safe to breast-feed
- Advise her that she can eat and drink within 1 hour of birth
- Monitor the baby's blood sugars
- In type 1 diabetics, Insulin requirements drop after delivery (put on a sliding scale and start a pre-pregnancy dose as soon as she starts eating)
- In type 2, recommence oral hypoglycaemics
- Advise the woman on contraception
  - Progestogen-only contraceptives are associated with an earlier onset of type 2 diabetes in women with previous gestational diabetes

- the combined oral contraceptive pill does not have this effect and may be used for women who are not breastfeeding
  - consider the Mirena intra-uterine device for contraception

Gestational Diabetes Mellitus (GDM)

- Prevalence varies from 9-20% depending on the population
- It is usually asymptomatic and develops in the second or third trimester
- It is more common if:
  - the maternal age ≥ 40 years
  - there is a family history of diabetes, especially a first degree relative
  - GDM was present in a previous pregnancy
  - BMI ≥ 30kg/m^2
  - they have had a previous baby weighing > 4.5kg
  - they have had a previous unexplained stillbirth, neonatal death or congenital malformation
  - they have polycystic ovary syndrome
  - it is a multiple pregnancy

Screening and diagnosis

- Recommend a 75g OGTT at 26-28 weeks for all pregnant women
  - for women with the above risk factors and taking into account ethnicity
    - recommend OGTT in the first trimester and repeat it at 26-28 weeks if initially normal – abnormal levels are:
      - fasting ≥ 5.1mmol/l
      - 1 hour ≥ 10.0mmol/l
      - 2 hours ≥ 8.5mmol/l
    - $HbA1_c$ ≥ 41mmol/l (5.9%) is abnormal in early pregnancy

Maternal risks

- Some women may have pre-existing diabetes and thus be prone to the same complications as type 2 diabetics
- There is increased risk of pre-eclampsia
- There is a higher incidence of macrosomia, especially if obese
- There is increased risk of a UTI, respiratory infections, endometritis and SSIs

- She may have polyhydramnios (associated with poor control and may lead to malpresentation, unstable lie and preterm labour)
- There is a higher risk of caesarean section
- There is higher risk of postpartum haemorrhage
- 50% will eventually become diabetic within 15 years following pregnancy and lifestyle changes may delay this

Fetal risks

- Macrosomia is associated with higher rates of neonatal morbidity (shoulder dystocia, severe hypoglycaemia, neonatal jaundice and brachial plexus injury)
- There is a risk of respiratory distress syndrome due to delayed lung maturation

Antenatal management

- Most of the care is similar to that for known diabetes in pregnancy
- Recommend blood tests as above
- Recommend Aspirin and Calcium as above
- Advise that the woman monitor glucose levels at home
    - aim for fasting levels of < 5.1mmol/l
    - 1 hour after commencement of meal < 7.4mmol/l
    - 2 hours after commencement of meal < 6.7mmol/l

- Provide advice on optimal weight gain in pregnancy
- The woman may require oral hypoglycaemic drugs (use metformin or glyburide)
- 15% of women will require Insulin and its use reduces the risk of macrosomia
    - recommend Insulin if
        - fasting blood sugar levels remain > 5.5mmol/l more than once a week
        - 1 hour post prandial level is > 6.7mmol/l on 2 or more occasions within a week regardless of diet

Timing of delivery

- If well controlled GDM on diet alone
    - await spontaneous labour
    - recommend IOL at 41^0-41^6 weeks as for post dates
- If well controlled GDM on metformin alone
    - recommend IOL at 39^0-39^6 weeks

Mode of delivery

- If scan EFW is > 4500g recommend an elective caesarean section

Management in labour

- Monitor hourly glucose and commence insulin/glucose infusion if its level ≥ 8 on two occasions
    - maintain levels 4-7mmol/l

Follow up postpartum

- Following delivery of the placenta cease any Insulin or oral hypoglycaemic agents
- Recommend a normal diet following delivery
- Assess diabetic control once she has resumed normal diet
- Repeat GTT and HbA1c 6-8 weeks after delivery
- If sugars remain consistently > 10mmol/L, this implies ongoing diabetes
    - treat as diabetic with physician
- Review by GP and discuss plans for counselling for future pregnancy

Recurrence

- One to two thirds of the women will develop GDM in a subsequent pregnancy
    - the risk is reduced if they adopt a lifestyle change and lose weight
- They have an increased risk of developing type 2 diabetes later in life (the risk being especially increased if they are obese)
    - a Progesterone only pill increases the risk of developing type 2 diabetes (use with caution)

Protocol for Insulin during labour

1. Type 1 Diabetes Mellitus

Induction of labour with Prostaglandin E2/balloon

- Continue with usual doses of Insulin until she is in established labour
- Administer a normal dose of long acting Insulin the night before induction
    - if the woman is on a morning dose of long acting Insulin, discuss dosage with the medical team

- o if she is on short acting Insulin continue until she is in established labour

Mainline cannula

- 1L 4% dextrose in normal saline (run at 80ml per hour)

Sideline

- 50 Units Actrapid in 0.9% normal saline made up to 50ml in a 50ml syringe (1 unit/ml solution)
    - o monitor blood glucose levels hourly on Insulin dependent diabetics
    - o monitor glucose levels 2 hourly if she is well controlled on diet alone

Infusion rate

- These are guidelines only and may need to be adjusted according to the glucose level

Blood glucose level (mmol/l)	**Insulin infusion (U/hour)**
4	Continue infusion and notify medical team
4.1-6.0	1
6.1-8.0	2
8.1-10	3
> 10	Notify and review by med team

- Aim for a blood glucose level between 4-7mmol/L
- Recommend the ward test urine every 2 hours
    - o notify medical team if there is > trace of ketonuria

Induction of labour with amniotomy or Syntocinon

- Continue using the usual dose of short and long acting Insulin until she is in established labour or if on nil orally
- Prior to commencement of induction, insert an intravenous cannula and commence infusions as above

Spontaneous labour

- Commence Insulin and dextrose/saline as above

Caesarean section

- Continue with the usual dose of short and long acting Insulin until she is nil by mouth and:
  - o insert an intravenous cannula with a mainline infusion of dextrose/saline solution
  - o commence Insulin infusion as above if glucose level is > 7mmol/L

Postpartum management
Vaginal birth

- Cease insulin infusion immediately following delivery unless blood sugar level (BGL) is > 10mmol/L
- Cease intravenous fluids unless BGL is < 4mmol/L or unable to tolerate diet
- Monitor BGL four times a day

Caesarean section

- Cease Insulin infusion immediately following delivery unless BGL is > 10mmol/L
- Continue sodium chloride 0.9% (1 litre) every 12 hours until tolerating diet (if on Syntocinon infusion for postpartum haemorrhage prevention use sodium chloride 0.9% after the Syntocinon infusion has ceased)
- Monitor BGL two hourly for 8 hours and then four times a day (pre-meals and pre-bed) until discharged
- Recommence Insulin therapy if BGL is > 10mmol/L
  - o if the woman is able to tolerate her diet, administer Insulin subcutaneously
  - o if nil by mouth or unable to tolerate diet, administer Insulin by intravenous infusion with dextrose/saline (1 litre every 12 hours)

2. Type 2 Diabetes Mellitus and Insulin treated Gestational Diabetes Mellitus

Induction of labour with Prostaglandin E2

- Advise an early morning breakfast and the usual dose of subcutaneous short acting Insulin
- Omit long acting Insulin
- Monitor BGL two hourly from 0700
- Commence Insulin and dextrose 4% / sodium chloride 0.18% infusion if BGL > 7mmol/l

Induction of labour with amniotomy or Syntocinon

- Advise an early morning breakfast and the usual dose of subcutaneous short acting Insulin
- Omit long acting Insulin
- Monitor BGL every two hours from 0700
- Commence Insulin and dextrose/saline infusion if BGL is > 7mmol/

Caesarean section

- Continue usual dose of short and long acting Insulin until the night before
- Advise nil by mouth from midnight
- Advise not taking subcutaneous insulin on the morning of the caesarean section
- Monitor BGL every 2 hours from 0700
- Commence Insulin and dextrose/sodium infusion if BGL is > 7mmol/L

Spontaneous labour

- Monitor BGL on arrival and then every 2 hours
- Commence Insulin and dextrose/saline infusion if BGL > 7mmol/L

Postpartum management
Vaginal birth

- If the woman commenced on an Insulin infusion then cease this immediately following delivery unless BGL is > 10mmol/L
- Cease intravenous fluids unless BGL is < 4mmol/L or she is unable to tolerate diet
- Commence BGL six hourly as a minimum (pre-meals and pre-bed)

Caesarean section

- If a woman commenced on an Insulin infusion then cease this immediately following delivery unless BGL is > 10mmol/L
- Commence normal saline (1 litre 12 hourly) if she is unable to tolerate her diet
- Monitor BGL every two hours for 8 hours and then four times daily (pre-meals and pre-bed) until she is discharged

Recommended Reading

1. Diabetes in pregnancy: management from preconception to the postnatal period. NICE guideline Published: 25 February 2015 nice.org.uk/guidance/ng3 https://www.nice.org.uk/Guidance/cg63
2. Berger H, Gagnon R, Sermer M et al. Diabetes in Pregnancy. *J. Obstet. Gynaecol. Can.* 2016; 38(7): 667-679.
3. American Diabetic association. Management of diabetes in pregnancy. *Diabetes Care*. 2015 Jan; 38 Suppl: S77-9.
4. Blumer I, Hadar E, Hadden DR et al. Diabetes and pregnancy: an endocrine society clinical practice guideline. *J. Clin. Endocrinol. Metab.* 2013 Nov; 98(11): 4227-49.
5. Catherine Nelson-Piercy. Diabetes mellitus, in *Handbook of Obstetric Medicine*, 2015; 5th Edition, CRC Press, pp. 85-101.

CHAPTER NINETEEN

EPILEPSY IN PREGNANCY

Effect of pregnancy on epilepsy

- Most women with controlled epilepsy have a normal pregnancy and outcome
- In about 30% of women seizure frequency may deteriorate, mostly due to poor compliance or sleep deprivation
    - the risk of seizure is highest during labour, at 1-2%
- Women who have been seizure free for 12 months or more have a lower risk of deterioration
- Drug levels are affected due to poor absorption and haemodilution of pregnancy

Effect of epilepsy on pregnancy

- Obstetric complications associated with epilepsy include:
    - fetal abnormality – dysmorphic features
        - this is more common with use of Valproate
    - trauma from seizures resulting in miscarriage or placental abruption
    - preterm labour
    - low birth weight
    - frequent seizure activity, which may result in episodes of hypoxaemia affecting fetal growth
    - the use of Valproate and other antiepileptic drugs, which may affect intellectual development of the newborn later in life

Management

Pre-pregnancy

- Inform women that risk of oral contraceptive failure is increased with enzyme-inducing antiepileptics:
    - Phenobarbitone, Phenytoin, Carbamazepine and Primidone
- Inform women of the importance of seizure control

- Recommend a periconceptual Folic acid 5mg / day supplementation to reduce the risk of folic acid deficiency induced malformations, especially with valproate and phenytoin
- Discuss the possibility of epilepsy occurring in offspring – offer genetic counselling if both parents are epileptic
- Optimise the treatment regimen six months prior to planned conception
- If a woman has had no seizures for 2 years consider tapering or ceasing treatment about six months before becoming pregnant
- Use a single drug with the lowest possible dose to minimise risk of teratogenicity
    - polytherapy may be associated with the greater risk of malformations

Antenatal

- See pregnant women with epilepsy with the physician in each trimester throughout pregnancy and document seizure frequency
- Avoid making changes to the treatment regimen for the purpose of reducing teratogenic risk in established pregnancy
- The goal of therapy is to maintain seizure control using the lowest effective antiepileptic drug (AED) dose
- In women with good control, there is no need to measure drug level in each trimester
- Avoid use of Valproate if possible
    - it appears that lamotrigine may be the first choice in women of childbearing age
- Recommend a morphology scan at 18 to 20 weeks to evaluate for neural tube defects, cleft lip and palate, and heart anomalies
- If women present with seizures in the second half of pregnancy without definitive diagnosis of epilepsy
    - follow existing protocols for eclampsia management until a definitive diagnosis is made by a full neurological assessment
    - consider other cardiac, metabolic and intracranial conditions in the differential diagnosis
    - consider also neuropsychiatric conditions
- Current evidence demonstrates not to recommend oral (10mg) vitamin K supplementation for women with epilepsy receiving AEDs in late pregnancy
    - recommend 1mg Vitamin K to the neonate
- Recommend induction of labour or caesarean section only for obstetric reasons

Intrapartum management

- There is an increased risk of seizure recurrence in labour and delivery; this may be due to
    - poor bioavailability of AEDs
    - noncompliance with medication
    - sleep deprivation
    - anxiety and hyperventilation during labour
- Ensure she has adequate analgesia to minimise pain and stress
- Ensure she has intravenous access and adequate hydration
- Continue oral anticonvulsants
    - if a dose is missed for more than 12 hours, it may be necessary to give her a parenteral dose
        - consult a physician or neurologist
    - if on oral phenytoin
        - continue the same dose intravenously in divided doses
    - if on any other anticonvulsant
        - recommend a Phenytoin loading dose (15-20mg/kg) with maintenance doses of 8mg/kg per day

Immediately following birth

- Recommend intramuscular Vitamin K_1 to the baby at birth
    - 1.0mg for term babies
    - 0.5mg for babies whose weight is < 1.5 kg
- If the mother requests an oral dose, administer 3 doses of 2.0mg:
    - at birth, on days 3-5 and at 4 weeks
- Monitor the baby closely for signs of respiratory depression – Valproate may be associated with jitteriness
- Examine the baby for any dysmorphic features

Postnatal

- Continue antiepileptic drugs and beware recurrence of seizures – consider changing dose to pre-pregnancy levels on day 10
- Advise that it is safe to breast-feed
- For contraception, recommend high dose combined OC with at least 50mcg Oestrogen to minimise breakthrough bleeding and failures or use Depo Provera
    - an oral Progestogen-only pill or Progesterone implants are unreliable if on enzyme-inducing anticonvulsants
    - the Levonorgestrel intrauterine device (IUD) (Mirena) is a useful contraceptive for these women

Recommended Reading

1. Ahmed R, Apen K and Endean C. Epilepsy in pregnancy. A collaborative team effort of obstetricians, neurologists and primary care physicians for a successful outcome. *Aust. Fam. Physician* 2014; 43(3): 110-114.
2. Battino D, Tomson T, Bonizzoni E et al. EURAP Study Group. Seizure control and treatment changes in pregnancy: observations from the EURAP epilepsy pregnancy registry. *Epilepsia* 2013; 54: 1621–7.
3. Borthen I, Eide MG, Daltveit AK et al. Obstetric outcome in women with epilepsy: a hospital-based, retrospective study. BJOG 2011;118: 956–65.
4. RCOG. Green-top Guideline No. 68 Epilepsy in pregnancy. June 2016.

CHAPTER TWENTY

FETAL GROWTH RESTRICTION

Small for gestational age (SGA) is defined as an estimated fetal weight of < 10th centile. Not all SGA babies have fetal growth restriction (FGR). 70% of babies that are SGA are constitutionally small due to female sex, ethnicity and BMI.

- With FGR the fetus has failed to achieve its growth potential
- Not all babies who have FGR are SGA

FGR- Delphi consensus definition

- Early (< 32weeks)
    - abdominal circumference (AC) or estimated fetal weight (EFW) is < 3rd centile or there is absent uterine artery end diastolic flow (UA-AEDF) **OR**
        - AC or EFW is < 10th centile **combined with**
        - uterine artery or umbilical artery (UA) pulsatility index (PI) > 95th centile
- Late (≥ 32weeks)
    - AC or EFW is < 3rd centile **OR**
        - at least **two** of the following:
            - AC or EFW < 10th centile
            - AC or EFW crossing centiles (> 2 quartiles on growth centiles)
            - cerebro-placental ration (CPR) is < 5th centile OR UA PI is > 95th centile

Diagnosis

Fundal height (FH) measurement

- It has poor sensitivity (25%), especially in women with high BMI
- Recommend measuring FH at each visit from 24-26 weeks and PLOT on fundal height chart
    - encourage the woman to empty her bladder if she has not done so in the last 30 minutes

  - position the woman in a supine position with a slight lateral tilt
  - identify the top of the fundus by gentle palpation
  - hold tape with the cm marking hidden and measure from the uppermost border of the uterine fundus to the uppermost border of the symphysis pubis, without applying pressure over the fundus
  - turn over the tape to read the measurement and record FH to the nearest cm
  - recommend a growth scan if:
    - there is single abnormal reading more than 3cm below/above the expected value
    - two successive readings are below/above the expected level
    - there is an abnormal trend
- Judicious use of FH charts doubles the chance of detecting FGR in nulliparous women

First trimester screen

- A low PAPP-A level (< 0.4 MOM) is a risk factor for subsequent FGR

Uterine artery doppler

- In high risk cases a uterine artery doppler at 20-22 weeks may predict subsequent development of FGR

Ultrasound scan for fetal biometry

- Serial measurements and observing growth velocity are more useful than looking at a single reading
  - always plot AC, head circumference (HC) and EFW on a growth chart and see the trend over 2 readings to differentiate SGA from FGR
  - estimation of liquor volume
    - use deepest pool of at least 2cmas being normal
    - amniotic fluid index of 6 or more as normal can also be used

Middle cerebral artery (MCA) doppler

- It provides information about the hemodynamic status of the fetus
  - in preterm FGR it is a poor indicator of adverse outcome
    - it should not be used to time delivery

  - in term FGR with normal uterine artery dopplers, an MCA doppler allows a moderate prediction for fetal acidaemia
    - MCA peak systolic velocity (PSV) of > 1.5 MOM or an increasing trend is abnormal

Ductus venosus doppler

It is a useful test to delay very preterm delivery in fetuses with absent or reversed end-diastolic arterial flow in the umbilical artery and a reassuring CTG

- It is not of much value in near term FGR

Cerebroplacental ratio (CPR)

- Calculate it by dividing MCA PI by UA PI. Generally, a CPR > 1:1 is normal
- CPR may predict a caesarean section for intrapartum fetal compromise in low risk pregnancies at term
- It may predict an adverse perinatal outcome in compromised fetuses regardless of fetal size
- It may be a marker of impaired fetal growth velocity even in fetuses whose size is considered appropriate using conventional biometry
- It is not of value in predicting the timing of birth – an umbilical artery doppler is more valuable for this purpose

Management

SGA

- Recommend continuing to perform 2-4 weekly scans to confirm growth remains along the centile
  - recommend delivery at 39 - 40 weeks

FGR

- Once a diagnosis of FGR is made, recommend monitoring for fetal wellbeing
  - recommend a weekly umbilical artery PI and CTG
  - recommend this twice weekly if there are other risk factors for stillbirth (SB)
    - aim to continue monitoring till delivery at about 38 weeks
    - deliver at 37 weeks if there are other risk factors for SB (HT, Previous SGA)

- an MCA doppler is usually of little value in the absence of FGR
- an MCA doppler is less reliable than an umbilical artery doppler in planning care

Other management considerations in general

- Advise them to stop smoking if they currently do so
- Recommend low dose of Aspirin, 150mg at night, from early in the first trimester in high risk cases
- If FGR is detected at the morphology scan
    - consider karyotyping
    - screen for CMV and Toxoplasmosis infection

The aim is to deliver the most mature fetus in the best possible condition before it develops fetal acidaemia or chronic hypoxia.

Recommended Reading

1. Salomon LJ, Alfirevic Z, Da Silva Costa F et al. Practice Guidelines: ultrasound assessment of fetal biometry and growth, *Ultrasound Obstet. Gynecol.* 2019; 53: 715–723.
2. Martins JG, Biggio TG and Abuhamad A. Society for Maternal-Fetal Medicine (SMFM) Consult Series #52: Diagnosis and Management of Fetal Growth 2019.
3. McCowan L, Figueras F, Anderson NH. Evidence-based national guidelines for the management of suspected fetal growth restriction: *Amer. J. Obstet. & Gynecol.* 2018.
4. Martins JG, Biggio JR, Abuhamad A. Society for Maternal-Fetal Medicine Consult Series #52: Diagnosis and management of fetal growth restriction. *Am. J. Obstet. Gynecol.* 2020 Oct; 223(4): B2-B1.
5. Verfaille V, de Jonge A, Mokkink L et al. Multidisciplinary consensus on screening for, diagnosis and management of fetal growth restriction in the Netherlands. BMC Pregnancy Childbirth. 2017 Oct 16; 17(1): 353. doi: 10.1186/s12884-017-1513-3.

CHAPTER TWENTY-ONE

FETAL WELLBEING – ANTEPARTUM ASSESSMENT

1. Fetal Movements (see Chapter on Decreased Fetal Movements)

2. FGR - See Chapter on Fetal Growth Restriction

3. Fetal Heart Rate Monitoring – Antenatal - NST/CTG

- A non-stress test (NST), often referred to as antenatal cardiotocography (CTG), is used as a useful adjunct to the care of women whose babies are at risk of hypoxia and or acidosis

Indications for CTG include:

- Preterm uterine activity
- Detection of fetal bradycardia or tachycardia
- Maternal perception of reduced fetal movements after 28 weeks
- Trauma to the abdomen (directly after)
- Pre and post external cephalic version
- Pre and post administration of mechanical and chemical cervical ripening agents
- Any other obstetric condition that increases the risk of fetal compromise

Procedure – A few points to note

- Ensure paper speed is set at 1cm per minute
- Cease monitoring as soon as all criteria for a normal test are met
    - if not, continue CTG for up to 90 minutes
- Avoid performing the test immediately after the woman has smoked a cigarette

Parameters

- Baseline fetal heart rate (FHR)
    - determine over 5-10 minutes
    - assess during a segment of trace in between contractions and fetal movements
    - normal baseline FHR is 110-160 beats/min (bpm)
- Baseline variability (BLV)
    - assess variation of the heart rate around the baseline
    - normal BLV is 6-25 bpm
        - view in a segment of trace in the absence of uterine contractions or fetal movements
            - reduced BLV is 3-5 bpm and absent BLV is < 3 bpm
- Reactivity
    - look for the presence of accelerations in response to movements
        - an acceleration is a rise in FHR of at least 15 bpm from baseline lasting for at least 15 secs
            - reactivity is normal if there are at least 2 accelerations in a 20 min period
            - if not, then continue CTG for up to 90 minutes
                - the fetus may be in a 'sleep mode' when accelerations may not be seen
                - this almost never lasts for more than 90 minutes
        - in pregnancies of less than 30 weeks gestation, an acceleration is defined as 10 bpm for 10 secs
- Decelerations
    - a normal trace should not have any decelerations

Normal CTG

- This indicates a fetus that is currently in good health. This is a trace where all 4 features are reassuring – a normal baseline, normal baseline variability, at least 2 accelerations in 20 mins and no decelerations

Non-reactive NST

- This is a trace with a normal baseline and normal baseline variability but no accelerations or decelerations. If the trace remains non-reactive after 60 min
    - repeat after 4 hours, **or**
    - try vibroacoustic stimulation – place the vibroacoustic source on or just above the maternal abdomen
        - this decreases the mean overall testing time by almost seven minutes and reduces the frequency of nonreactive CTGs by 40 percent

Abnormal trace

- This is a trace that shows decelerations (these require careful assessment especially where there is FGR); shallow prolonged decelerations are very concerning

Sinusoidal pattern

- This is a CTG with a smooth, undulating pattern of 2-5 cycles per minute with an amplitude of 5-15 bpm, lasting at least 10 minutes. They often have an absent baseline variability and usually no accelerations
- A pseudo sinusoidal pattern resembles sinusoidal features, but with a more jagged 'saw-tooth' appearance. Its duration seldom exceeds 30 minutes and is characterised by normal features, before and after

Recommended Reading

1. The Royal Australian and New Zealand College of Obstetricians and Gynaecologists (2014) Intrapartum Fetal Surveillance Clinical Guidelines – fourth edition 2019.
2. Baker L, Beaves M, and Wallace E. 2016. Assessing Fetal Wellbeing A Practical Guide. Southern Health and RANZCOG. 2016.
3. Shrestha S, Shrestha I. Admission Cardiotocography in Predicting Perinatal Outcome. *Kathmandu Univ. Med. J. (KUMJ)*. 2019 Jul-Sept.;17(67):201-205.
4. Lear CA, Westgate JA, Ugwumadu A et al. Understanding Fetal Heart Rate Patterns That May Predict Antenatal and Intrapartum Neural Injury. *Semin. Pediatr. Neurol.* 2018 Dec; 28: 3-16.
5. Simpson L, Khati NJ, Deshmukh SP et al. ACR Appropriateness Criteria Assessment of Fetal Well-Being. *J. Am. Coll. Radiol.* 2016 Dec; 13(12 Pt A): 1483-1493.

CHAPTER TWENTY-TWO

FETAL WELLBEING – INTRAPARTUM ASSESSMENT

Fetal Heart Rate

See also chapter on "Fetal wellbeing - Antepartum assessment"

- Not all fetal heart rate (FHR) abnormalities in labour are associated with fetal distress
- Use of continuous electronic FHR monitoring in labour by itself increases the rate of caesarean section (CS) and operative vaginal delivery
- Some data suggest that there may be benefits from the use of Sildenafil in labour in reducing risk of CS for fetal distress

Normal FHR

- Baseline FHR is 110-160 bpm
- Baseline variability is 6-25 bpm
- There may be accelerations
- There are no decelerations

Early decelerations

- There is uniform gradual decrease in FHR before or with a contraction and it returns to normal before the end of the contraction – it is a mirror image of the contraction curve
    - it is usually associated with head compression

Simple variable decelerations

- These are decelerations usually of rapid onset and with a rapid recovery that have little or no relationship with contractions and vary in depth and duration
    - there may be shouldering – this indicates a good fetal response
        - loss of shouldering may indicate loss of autonomic control
    - these are usually associated with cord compression

Complicated variable decelerations

- These have in addition a rising baseline or fetal tachycardia > 160 bpm, reduced variability with loss of shouldering, delay in returning to normal baseline, a drop by 60 bpm or drop to 60 bpm, or last for 60 sec or more
    - this pattern is more likely to be associated with hypoxia

Late decelerations

- These are uniform, repetitive decreases of FHR, usually starting from the middle to end of a contraction, with a nadir that is more than 20 seconds after the peak of the contraction
    - the longer the lag time the more likely this is associated with hypoxia

Prolonged deceleration

- There is a drop in baseline to less than 100 bpm lasting for > 90 secs but for < 5 mins

Fetal bradycardia

- There is a drop in baseline to less than 100 bpm lasting for > 5 mins

Terminology

- **Normal (green)**
    - normal baseline, normal variability and no decelerations
- **Abnormal unlikely (blue)**
    - baseline of 100-109 with early or variable decelerations and no accelerations
- **Abnormal may be (yellow)**
    - baseline tachycardia of > 160 bpm, rising baseline, reduced variability (3-5 bpm for > 30 min), complicated variable or late decelerations
- **Abnormal likely (red)**
    - bradycardia for > 5 min, absent variability (< 3bpm) for > 30 min, sinusoidal pattern, complicated variable decelerations with reduced or absent variability or late decelerations with reduced or absent variability or 2 or more features defined as abnormal likley

ST waveform analysis of the fetal electrocardiogram

- use of this has shown to significantly reduce metabolic acidosis and operative vaginal delivery rates compared with cardiotocography alone

Management of FHR abnormality

- Assess the whole picture – take account of current and past pregnancies, progress and stage of labour and type of FHR abnormality
- Identify any reversible cause and initiate appropriate action
    - turn the woman on her side
    - stop Syntocinon, if she's on it
    - administer 250mcg Terbutaline subcutaneously if she's contracting or has tachysystole
    - administer 1L normal saline rapidly

Fetal blood sampling (FBS)

- Common indications for FBS include:
    - fetal bradycardia
    - complicated tachycardia
    - recurrent decelerations
    - prolonged episodes of bradycardia or undefined deceleration patterns
    - prolonged loss of variability which does not spontaneously correct with fetal stimulation
    - other non-specific concerns about fetal wellbeing
- Only 50% of fetuses with baseline tachycardia and late decelerations will actually be acidotic at birth
- Lack of confirmation with FBS may result in unnecessary intervention
- When interpreting the result of FBS consider again previous results, progress of labour and any other clinical circumstances
- Contraindications to FBS include:
    - maternal blood borne infections such as HIV infection, sero-positive hepatitis (RNA positive) and active genital HSV infection
    - confirmed or suspected fetal bleeding disorders (haemophilia, low platelet count)
    - preterm (less than 34^0 weeks)
    - fetal malpresentation such as breech
    - or if any delay in expediting birth is contraindicated

Procedure

- A lateral position is preferable – if the lithotomy position is used, ensure there is a lateral tilt (use a wedge)
- Attach the fetal scalp blade to an introducer
- Insert an amnioscope with a light source if available
- Position the amnioscope onto the fetal scalp
- Clean the fetal scalp surface with chlorhexidine
- Clean it with a dry cotton wool swab
- Apply sterile liquid paraffin onto the fetal scalp to help with droplet formation
- Stab the scalp with the blade and use a heparinised capillary tube to collect blood by capillary action
- Test the sample as soon as possible
- Apply pressure with a swab onto the fetal scalp for a few minutes to stop bleeding from the puncture site

Fetal scalp pH values

- pH > 7.25 or lactate ≤ 4.1 is normal
    - if CTG then returns to normal there is no need to repeat
    - if not recommend a repeat in 1 hour or earlier if there is deterioration and delivery is not indicted
- pH 7.21-7.24 or lactate 4.2-4.8 is termed pre-acidotic
    - recommend repeat FBS in 30 minutes
    - if there is a rapid drop from previous sample, consider immediate delivery
- pH < 7.20 or lactate > 4.8 indicates fetal acidemia
    - recommend immediate delivery

Cord blood sampling at birth - Paired cord blood sampling at birth

Recommended indications include:

- All cases of emergency caesarean section
- Small for gestational age - baby < 10th centile
- Fetal growth restriction
- Multiple pregnancy
- Preterm birth < 37 weeks gestation
- Any significant fetal heart rate abnormality
- Intrapartum fever (≥ 38°C)
- Instrumental delivery
- Vaginal breech delivery
- Shoulder dystocia

Can cord blood analysis with delayed cord clamping

- Generally, restrict delayed cord clamping to vigorous healthy infants
- Avoid delayed cord clamping when prompt newborn resuscitation is indicated
- When cord clamping is delayed, samples of umbilical arterial and venous blood for gas analysis can still be obtained by drawing the samples from the pulsating, unclamped cord immediately after birth
- This procedure appears to be safe and has no effect on either the accuracy of the gas analysis or the volume of transfusion that the infant receives
- If a blood specimen for acid-base testing is desired after delayed cord clamping has been completed, a delay of up to two minutes appears to have no or only a small effect on the results
- It is generally accepted that arterial and venous pH should differ by 0.03 to be sure that the artery and vein have been sampled
- A pH of < 7.20 may result in significant short and long-term outcomes for the newborn

Recommended Reading

1. Dore S, Ehman W. No. 396-Fetal Health Surveillance: Intrapartum Consensus Guideline. *J. Obstet. Gynaecol. Can.* 2020 Mar; 42(3): 316-348.
2. Dawson JA, Schmölzer GM, Wyllie J. Monitoring heart rate in the delivery room. *Semin. Fetal Neonatal Med.* 2018 Oct; 23(5): 327-332.
3. Liston R, Sawchuck D, Young D. No. 197b-Fetal Health Surveillance: Intrapartum Consensus Guideline. *J. Obstet. Gynaecol. Can.* 2018 Apr; 40(4): e298-e322.
4. The Royal Australian and New Zealand College of Obstetricians and Gynaecologists (2014) Intrapartum Fetal Surveillance Clinical Guidelines - Fourth Edition 2019.
5. West S, Ibiebele I, Nippita T. Intrapartum fetal blood sampling performed at early cervical dilatation and delivery outcomes. *Aust. N. Z. J. Obstet. Gynaecol.* 2021 Jun; 61(3): 403-407.
6. Lear CA, Westgate JA, Ugwumadu A et al. Understanding Fetal Heart Rate Patterns That May Predict Antenatal and Intrapartum Neural Injury. *Semin. Pediatr. Neurol.* 2018 Dec; 28: 3-16.
7. Raghuraman N, Cahill AG. Update on Fetal Monitoring: Overview of Approaches and Management of Category II Tracings. *Obstet. Gynecol. Clin. North Am.* 2017 Dec; 44(4): 615-624.

CHAPTER TWENTY-THREE

FIBROIDS IN PREGNANCY

Effect of the pregnancy on fibroids

- Traditional teaching is that fibroids increase in size during pregnancy but several studies have shown that there is no consistent change in size and some may even get smaller
- If they increase in size most do so in the first trimester

Effect of fibroids on the pregnancy

- Submucosal fibroids increase the risk of miscarriages, bleeding and subfertility, especially if they distort the uterine cavity
- Fibroids can cause pain, especially if they are > 5cm in diameter. They present often in the second and third trimesters and are due to red degeneration or torsion if the fibroid is pedunculated
- They can cause malpresentation and or obstruction in labour
- Placental abruption can occur especially if they are located close to the placental site
- FGR
- Preterm labour
- Increased risk of CS
- Retained placenta
- Postpartum haemorrhage

Management

Pre pregnancy

- Recommend at least a 6-month interval between myomectomy and subsequent conception

Antenatal

- Recommend iron supplementation to minimise risk of anaemia
    - this may avoid blood transfusion if she has a postpartum haemorrhage (PPH)

- also discuss use of cell saver
- Pain management (Ibuprofen is mostly used)
  - if using NSAIDS for pain, recommend using it for no more than 48 hours
- Recommend surgery if
  - there is uncontrollable pain
  - they increase in size rapidly
  - a fibroid larger than 5cm is present in the lower segment
    - the best time to operate is in the first and second trimesters

Birth

- If the endometrium is encroached during a pre-pregnancy myomectomy, recommend an elective caesarean section (CS)
  - some say recommend CS even if < 50% of the myometrium is encroached
    - ensure the uterine incision is 2cm away from any fibroid
    - if at the time of CS a fibroid is seen in the lower segment, consider performing a classical CS
      - make classical CS incision at least 10cm long
      - consider the use of a cell saver
- If having a vaginal birth
  - recommend active management of the 3rd stage of labour with a Syntocinon bolus injection followed by an infusion for 24 hours if there are numerous fibroids
  - a balloon tamponade may also be required to control bleeding postpartum
- A myomectomy at the time of the caesarean section
  - contrary to previous beliefs, evidence now supports performing a myomectomy at the time of the CS
  - surgery at the time of CS is indicated:
    - if fibroids are causing difficulty with closure of the uterine incision
    - to facilitate safe delivery of the fetus
    - if they are large (greater than 6cm in diameter)
    - if there are sub serosal fibroids
      - myomectomy also increases the chance of future spontaneous conception

Postpartum

- Fibroids usually continue to regress for up to 3-6 months postpartum in over 70% of women
    - regression is faster in African women
    - it is slower if using Progesterone only contraception

Recommended Reading

1. Sampat K, Alleemudder DI. Fibroids in pregnancy: management and outcomes. *The Obstetrician Gynaecologist*; 2018; 20(3): 187-195
2. Lee HC, Norwitz ER and Shaw J. Contemporary Management of Fibroids in Pregnancy, *Rev. Obstet. Gynecol.* 2010; 3(1): 20–27.
3. Coutinho LM, Assis WA, Spagnuolo-Souza A, Reis FM. Uterine Fibroids and Pregnancy: How Do They Affect Each Other? *Reprod. Sci.* 2021 Jun 17. doi: 10.1007/s43032-021-00656-6.
4. Goyal M, Dawood AS, Elbohoty SB et al. Cesarean myomectomy in the last ten years; A true shift from contraindication to indication: A systematic review and meta-analysis. *Eur. J. Obstet. Gynecol. Reprod. Biol.* 2021 Jan; 256: 145-157.
5. Pérez-Roncero GR, López-Baena MT, Ornat L et al. Uterine fibroids and preterm birth risk: A systematic review and meta-analysis. *J. Obstet. Gynaecol. Res.* 2020 Sep; 46(9): 1711-1727.

CHAPTER TWENTY-FOUR

FIRST TRIMESTER SCREEN

Dating scan

- Accurate dating is important for the management of pregnancy
- An early ultrasound scan may also identify severe lethal malformations
    - anencephaly
    - cystic hygroma

First trimester screening for chromosomal abnormality

- Recommend combined first trimester screen (CFTS) for trisomy 13, 18 and 21. This includes a combination of:
    - nuchal translucency and serum Papp-A, serum beta hCG levels and maternal age
    - recommend scan at between 11^0 and 13^6 weeks gestation
    - recommend the blood test at any time between 10 and 13 weeks
        - increased NT ($\geq$ 3.5mm) is associated with an increased risk of cardiac abnormality and skeletal dysplasia.
        - low Papp-A (< 0.40 MoM):
            - it is associated with increased risk of chromosomal abnormality
            - it is also associated with increased risk of miscarriage, FGR, pre-eclampsia, preterm birth, placental abruption and stillbirth
                - offer a uterine artery doppler between 22 and 24 weeks
                - recommend regular growth scans
        - a level of 0.20 MoM or less is associated with Cornelia de Lange syndrome

- Recommend a first trimester triple test (combination of maternal factors and measurements of mean arterial blood pressure, uterine artery pulsatility index, and serum placental growth factor)
    - it is a good predictor of early onset preeclampsia and SGA, with a 10% false-positive rate
- recommend non-invasive prenatal testing (NIPT) from 10 weeks
    - it can identify 99% of babies with Down's Syndrome
    - it can also detect other chromosomal disorders
        - offer chorionic villus sampling or amniocentesis to confirm diagnosis

Second trimester anomaly scan

- Ultrasound scan at 18^0-20^6 weeks
    - assess fetal biometry, anatomy, amniotic fluid volume, placental position and also examine for any pathology in the maternal adnexa and cervical length
    - if placenta is low lying
        - recommend a repeat scan at 34 weeks
    - if you suspect any abnormality
        - refer the woman for a Maternal Fetal Medicine (MFM) scan
    - renal pelvis dilatation:
        - dilatation of $\geq$ 5mm at 18-26 weeks may be a marker for renal tract abnormality
        - it is not a useful marker for trisomy 21
            - if dilatation is < 10mm
                - no action is required antenatally
                - offer a neonatal scan 10-14 days after birth
            - if dilatation is $\geq$ 10mm
                - refer them for an MFM scan to exclude other abnormalities
    - hyperechogenic bowel
        - the fetal bowel appears as bright as the fetal bone
        - this may be associated with FGR, cystic fibrosis, chromosomal abnormality, CMV, Toxoplasma or Herpes infection

- absent nasal bone
  - it is associated with increased risk of trisomy 21
  - 1% of normal people have an absent nasal bone
  - prevalence is higher in some ethnic groups
    - recommend amniocentesis if the nasal bone is absent
- isolated echogenic cardiac focus and isolated choroid plexus cysts
  - both are of no significance if the CFTS result is low risk
- isolated single umbilical artery
  - this is of no clinical significance if the CFTS result is low risk
- short femur or humerus
  - this may be associated with chromosomal abnormality, FGR or skeletal dysplasia
  - offer a triple test if CFTS has not been performed
  - scan for FGR

Recommended Reading

1. Liao Y, Wen H, Ouyang S et al. Routine first-trimester ultrasound screening using a standardized anatomical protocol. *Am. J. Obstet. Gynecol.* 2020 Oct 27: S0002-9378(20)31267-9.
2. Papastefanou I, Wright D, Lolos M et al. Competing-risks model for prediction of small-for-gestational-age neonates from maternal characteristics, serum PAPP-A and PlGF at 11-13 weeks' gestation. *Ultrasound. Obstet. Gynecol.* 2020 Sep 16. doi: 10.1002/uog.23118.
3. Cordisco A, Periti E, Antoniolli N et al. Clinical implementation of pre-eclampsia screening in the first trimester of pregnancy. *Pregnancy Hypertens.* 2021 May 14; 25: 34-38.
4. Simula N, Brown R, Butt K et al. Committee Opinion No. 418: The Complete 11-14 Week Prenatal Sonographic Examination. *J. Obstet. Gynaecol.* Can. 2021 May 17: S1701-2163(21)00375-3.
5. Bedei I, Wolter A, Weber A et al. Chances and Challenges of New Genetic Screening Technologies (NIPT) in *Prenatal Medicine from a Clinical Perspective: A Narrative Review*. Genes (Basel). 2021 Mar 29; 12(4): 501.
6. Elfassy L, Lasry A, Gil Y, Balayla J. Prevalence threshold of screening tests in obstetrics and gynecology. *Eur. J. Obstet. Gynecol. Reprod. Biol.* 2021 Apr; 259: 191-195.

CHAPTER TWENTY-FIVE

GROUP B STREPTOCOCCAL INFECTION

10-30% of all women are colonised by group B streptococcus (GBS). It is the commonest cause of early onset neonatal sepsis, pneumonia, and meningitis.
Vaginal colonisation and GBS bacteriuria are risk factors for early onset GBS disease (EOGBSD).

- If untreated, 40–50% of babies born to GBS positive mothers will become colonised and of these 1-2% will become infected
- Risk factors for EOGBSD include:
    - preterm labour (PTL) < 37 weeks (spontaneous or induced)
    - prolonged rupture of membranes ≥ 18 hours prior to birth
    - maternal temperature ≥ 38 degrees Centigrade in labour
    - GBS colonisation in the current pregnancy
    - GBS bacteriuria in the current pregnancy (any colony count)
    - previous baby with EOGBSD
- Diagnosis is either by routine screening of all pregnant women or screening based on risk factors
    - there is no strong evidence to support one or the other

Diagnosis

- Universal screening involves performing a low vaginal and perianal swab at around 36 weeks in all pregnant women
- New US guidelines recommend screening for GBS at 36^0-37^6 weeks
    - they recommend re-testing GBS negative women 5 weeks later
        - if GBS is positive, recommend intrapartum antibiotics
        - if GBS is negative, recommend intrapartum antibiotics if her previous infant was affected by GBS infection or if she has had GBS bacteriuria at any stage in the current pregnancy
        - if GBS status is unknown, base management on presence of risk factors for EOGBSD

- if risk factors are present – recommend intrapartum antibiotics
- if they are absent, manage as normal

Management

- It is not recommended to treat the antenatal detection of GBS in the vagina or urine
    - treat a GBS urinary tract infection (UTI) at any gestation in the current pregnancy (usually where the quantitative count is greater than or equal to 10^5 cfu/m)
- Antibiotic prophylaxis is not recommended in the following circumstances
    - elective CS (no labour, no rupture of membranes) irrespective of GBS status or the gestational age
    - unknown GBS status without EOGBSD in a previous pregnancy
    - threatened preterm labour with intact membranes where the risk of imminent birth is low
    - prelabour rupture of membranes (ROM) at or near term but prior to the onset of labour (even if membranes have been ruptured for more than 18 hours)
        - recommend antibiotics once in labour or, if she is being induced, as soon as the duration of ROM reaches or exceeds 14 hours and birth is assessed as unlikely before duration of ROM equals 18 hours
- Recommend intrapartum antibiotics to women with the risk factors noted above

Choice of antibiotics

- Intravenous Benzylpenicillin 3g at the onset of labour and then 1.8g every 4 hours until birth
    - Erythromycin is not recommended due to increasing rates of antibiotic resistance
    - if she is allergic to Penicillin
        - recommend intravenous Lincomycin (or Clindamycin) 600mg every 8 hours until birth
    - if the maternal temperature $\geq 38^0$C intrapartum, recommend a triple antibiotic regime
        - Ampicillin (or Amoxicillin) 2g initially and then 2g every 6 hours

- Gentamicin 5mg/kg once daily
- Metronidazole 500mg every 12 hours
    - continue intravenous antibiotic treatment for 24 hours at least
    - recommend oral antibiotics once afebrile and tolerating oral medication
    - continue for up to 5 days total
- send fresh placenta to pathology

Recommended Reading

1. Williams M, Zantow E, Turrentine M. Cost Effectiveness of Latest Recommendations for Group B Streptococci Screening in the United States. *Obstet. Gynecol.* 2020 Apr; 135(4): 789-798.
2. Howard ED. Perinatal Management of Group B Streptococcal Infection: Clinical Update. *J. Perinat. Neonatal Nurs.* 2019 Oct/Dec; 33(4): 280-282.
3. Geethanath RM, Ahmed I, Abu-Harb M et al. Intrapartum antibiotics for prolonged rupture of membranes at term to prevent Group B Streptococcal sepsis. *J. Obstet. Gynaecol.* 2019 Jul; 39(5): 619-622.
4. Filkins L, Hauser JR, Robinson-Dunn B et al. American Society for Microbiology Provides 2020 Guidelines for Detection and Identification of Group B Streptococcus. *J. Clin. Microbiol.* 2020 Dec 17; 59(1): e01230-20.
5. Steer PJ, Russell AB, Kochhar S et al. Group B streptococcal disease in the mother and newborn-A review. *Eur. J. Obstet. Gynecol. Reprod. Biol.* 2020 Sep; 252: 526-533.

CHAPTER TWENTY-SIX

HEPATITIS C INFECTION IN PREGNANCY

The Hepatitis C virus is the primary cause of non-A non-B hepatitis. Hepatitis C is transmitted by sharing contaminated needles, needle stick injury, the transfusion of contaminated blood or blood products, and tattooing. Sexual transmission is rare. It is the commonest cause of post transfusion hepatitis although only 15% have a history of it. The commonest risk factor is intravenous drug use.

80% of those who are Hep C positive may develop chronic infection.

- 20% of these will develop cirrhosis of the liver
- They have an increased risk of developing obstetric cholestasis which may occur earlier than is usual

Antenatal management

- If the woman is a known Hepatitis C positive case
    - repeat to confirm she is still Hepatitis C antibody positive
- If she is Hepatitis C positive on routine screening in pregnancy
    - perform routine baseline liver function tests (LFTs) and request Hepatitis C RNA PCR at booking and repeat LFTs again at 28 weeks
        - if she is RNA negative: this may indicate a false positive antibody test, past cleared infection, past successful treatment, or low level viraemia below assay detection level
            - recommend testing the infant at 18 months of age
        - if she is RNA positive
            - the risk of perinatal transmission is 5%
- Scc thc woman at a joint clinic with a physician
- Encourage the mother to avoid alcohol, recreational drugs and smoking
- Counsel her about ways of reducing reinfection
- Recommend testing for Hepatitis B and human immunodeficiency virus (HIV) if she has not been tested

Labour

- Mode of birth
    - a caesarean section will reduce the risk of perinatal transmission even though this risk is only 5%
- Intrapartum care if planning vaginal birth
    - if she is RNA positive – avoid fetal scalp electrode and fetal blood sampling
- Ensure normal precautions when giving injections, taking blood, or performing vaginal examinations

Newborn

- Refer to a paediatrician for follow up
- Delay any injection until after bathing to remove any maternal blood on the baby
- It is safe to breast-feed; if she has cracked nipples, advise to express and discard milk until healed
- Arrange a single room with private toilet facilities following delivery
- Recommend testing the infant for Hep C RNA at 3 months
    - if negative – test Hep C antibody at 12-18 months
        - if still negative, infant has not been infected
    - if positive – request Hep C RNA and LFTs and refer to a specialist

Recommended Reading

1. Palasanthiran P, Starr M, Jones C, Eds.: *Management of perinatal infections*. Sydney: Australasian Society for Infectious Diseases (ASID); 2014.
2. Tagkou NM, Kondylis G, Cholongitas E. Pregnancy and Viral Hepatitis: Current Concepts. *Curr. Pharm. Des.* 2020 Dec 9. doi: 10.2174/1381612826666201210113841.
3. Chilaka VN, Konje JC. Viral Hepatitis in pregnancy. *Eur. J. Obstet. Gynecol. Reprod. Biol.* 2021 Jan; 256: 287-296.
4. Kushner T, Reau N. Changing epidemiology, implications, and recommendations for hepatitis C in women of childbearing age and during pregnancy. *J. Hepatol.* 2021 Mar; 74(3): 734-741.
5. Seto MT, Cheung KW, Hung IFN. Management of viral hepatitis A, C, D and E in pregnancy. *Best Pract. Res. Clin. Obstet. Gynaecol.* 2020 Oct; 68: 44-53.
6. Ragusa R, Corsaro LS, Frazzetto E et al. Hepatitis C Virus Infection in Children and Pregnant Women: An Updated Review of the Literature on Screening and Treatments. *AJP Rep.* 2020 Jan; 10(1): e121-e127.

CHAPTER TWENTY-SEVEN

HEPATITIS B INFECTION IN PREGNANCY

Perinatal transmission is the common form of transmission.

Hepatitis B virus (HBV) infection is mostly acquired through sexual transmission, via blood and body fluids.

Clinical features

- Symptoms of acute infection occur in 50% of cases
    - these include nausea, vomiting, fever, abdominal pain, dark stools and jaundice
- Chronic infection may result in cirrhosis of the liver or liver cancer
    - refer to an appropriate clinic for long term follow up
    - pregnant women have a 25% chance of dying from cirrhosis or liver cancer
- In pregnancy, 10-20% of women who are HBsAg positive will transmit the virus to the fetus in the absence of immune-prophylaxis
    - risk of transmission to the fetus is greatest if the mother is HBsAg and HBeAg positive
    - transmission mostly occurs at delivery
- If she is positive on routine screening for HBsAg, also recommend:
    - an HBeAg test
    - an HBeAb test
    - an HBV DNA test
    - LFTs
    - prothrombin time
    - a liver scan

Serology

- HBs Ag is the protein on the surface of the virus. It is found in acute and chronic cases. It is used to screen for infection
- The anti HBs antibody (ab) is a surface antibody and remains positive for life. It will also remain positive after successful vaccination

- The anti HBc ab IgM is only present in the liver and cannot be detected in blood. It indicates acute recent (< 6 months) infection
- HBe Antigen is produced in response to actively replication HBV – it is a marker of infectivity and is used to monitor effectiveness of treatment
- An anti HBe antibody is used to monitor recovery
- A high Hep B viral DNA count indicates an active multiplying virus and indicates that the person is infectious

Interpretation of results

- HBsAg negative, anti-HBc ab negative and anti-HBs ab negative; this indicates that she is susceptible to HBV infection and would benefit from being vaccinated if she is at high risk
- HBsAg positive, anti HBs ab negative, anti HBc ab (IgM and IgG) negative, HBe Ag positive and anti HBe ab negative; this indicates she has early acute infection and may still be asymptomatic
- HBsAg positive, anti-HBs ab negative, anti-HBc ab (IgM and IgG) positive or negative, anti-HBc IgM positive or negative, HBe positive and HBe ab negative; this indicates an acute infection and the woman will usually be symptomatic
- HBsAg positive, anti-HBs ab negative, anti-HBc (IgM and IgG) ab positive, HBc IgM ab positive, HBe Ag negative but HBe ab positive; this indicates an advanced acute phase of infection
- HBsAg positive, anti-HBs ab negative, anti-HBc (IgM and IgG) ab positive, anti-HBc IgM ab negative, HBe Ag positive but HBe ab negative; this indicates active chronic infection – liver damage cannot be excluded
- HBsAg positive, anti-HBs ab negative, anti-HBc (IgM and IgG) ab positive, anti-HBc IgM ab negative, HBe Ag negative but HBe ab positive; this indicates chronic infection and there is a low risk of liver damage
- HBsAg negative, anti-HBs positive, anti-HBc IgM and IgG ab negative; this indicates immunity to HBV due to hepatitis B vaccination
- HBsAg negative, anti-HBs ab negative anti-HBc IgM and IgG ab positive, HBe Ag negative and HBe ab positive; this indicates a resolving infection
- HBsAg negative, anti-HBs ab positive, anti HBc IgM negative, anti-HBc IgM and IgG ab positive, HBe Ag negative and HBe ab positive; this indicates a resolved infection and complete recovery

Management of pregnant woman exposed to Hep B infection

- Check her serology urgently
    - if anti-HBs ab level is > 10 IU/mL – take no action
        - vaccinate the infant at 2, 4 and 6 months
    - if anti-HBs ab level is < 10 IU/mL – recommend Hepatitis B vaccine and Hepatitis B immunoglobulin (HBIG) within 72 hours of exposure (administered at separate sites). Repeat vaccine at 1 and 6 months after the first dose
        - test mother for HBsAg again at 3 months
        - recommend HBIG and hepatitis B vaccine to newborn within 12 hours of birth

Management of woman who is HBsAg positive

- Discuss this with the woman as she may already be aware that she has a chronic infection
- If it is an acute infection consider counselling by appropriate staff
    - provide any written information available
    - test for Hep B viral DNA
        - if < 10^7 IU/ml
            - recommend HBIG and HB vaccination at birth
        - if > 10^7 IU/mL
            - refer her for treatment (Lamivudine or Tenofovir) from 30 weeks to reduce the risk of perinatal transmission
                - cease treatment 4-12 weeks postpartum
                    - check LFTS every 4 weeks for a few months for possible flare ups

Risks for baby

- Infants born to mothers who are HBsAg positive are vulnerable to infection and 90% become chronic carriers
    - 25% of infants who are chronic carriers will develop cirrhosis or hepatocellular cancer later in life

Labour

- There is no evidence that a caesarean section will prevent vertical transmission – thus it is not recommended

- During labour
    - minimise invasive procedures particularly in women with a high viral load although the magnitude of benefit in preventing perinatal transmission is uncertain – avoid FBS and FSE
- Ensure normal precautions when giving injections, taking blood or performing vaginal examinations

Newborn

- Delay any injection until after bathing and remove any maternal blood on the newborn baby
- Recommend HBIG within 12 hours of birth in one limb and monovalent Hep B vaccine at the same time in the other limb for the newborn – preferably within 7 days
- Repeat the vaccine at 2, 4 and 6 months of age
    - repeat testing for HBsAg and anti-HBc ab at age 9-12 months
        - if HBs Ag negative and anti-HBs ab level is < 10 IU/mL, consider further vaccine doses
        - if HBs Ag negative and anti-HBs ab level is > 10 IU/ml, no further action is required
        - if HBs Ag positive, refer for ongoing management
- It is safe to breast feed
- Arrange a single room with private toilet facilities for women following delivery

Follow up

- Check Hep B status of the partner and offer vaccination if the partner is non-immune

Recommended Reading

1. Palasanthiran P, Starr M, Jones C, editors. *Management of perinatal infections*. Sydney: Australasian Society for Infectious Diseases (ASID); 2014.
2. Yankowitz J and Pastorek II, Maternal and fetal viral infections. In: *High Risk Pregnancy* Eds. James DK, Steer PJ, Weiner CP and Gonik B. WB Saunders 45th Edition 2017. pp. 541-46.
3. Maraolo AE, Choosing the appropriate pharmacotherapy for hepatitis B during pregnancy: what are the considerations? *Expert Opin. Pharmacother*. 2021 Jun; 22(9): 1083-1086.

4. Chung EK, Enquobahrie DA. Perinatal Hepatitis B Prevention: Eliminating Disease and Disparity. *Pediatrics*. 2021 Mar; 147(3): e2020037549.
5. Perino J, Adams CN. The Importance of Hepatitis B Antigen Screening in Pregnancy. *Neonatal Netw.* 2020 Nov 1; 39(6): 363-368.
6. Sirilert S, Tongsong T. Hepatitis B Virus Infection in Pregnancy: An Update on Evidence-Based Management. *Obstet. Gynecol. Surv.* 2020 Sep; 75(9): 557-565.

CHAPTER TWENTY-EIGHT

HERPES SIMPLEX INFECTION IN PREGNANCY

5% of all women of childbearing age report a history of genital herpes.

90% of affected individuals are unaware as infection is often subclinical.

Both HSV 1 and HSV 2 can cause genital herpes – most cases of recurrent genital herpes are caused by HSV 2.

Due to increasing oral-genital contact, about 15% of genital HSV infections are due to HSV 1.

Primary infection

- 2% of women acquire primary genital HSV infection during pregnancy
    - if she is in the first trimester it increases the risk of early miscarriage
    - 85% of neonatal HSV infections are acquired prenatally
- Intrauterine infection accounts for < 5% of neonatal infections
- Lesions appear 2-14 days after exposure and may last for 20 days if not treated
    - lesions are painful and itchy and form ulcers when they rupture
    - there may be vaginal discharge
    - there may be fever malaise and local lymph node enlargement
- Although antibodies remain in the blood they do not prevent recurrences

Diagnosis

- HSV 1 IgG and HSV 2 IgG are negative but HSV - IgM is positive (either type 1 or 2)
- PCR from the genital tract will be positive
    - if they seroconvert < 30-34 weeks
        - risk of transmission is the same as for women with recurrent infection

- if they do not seroconvert
  - risk of transmission is high
    - 25-50%

Non-Primary first infection

- This is defined as previous confirmed exposure to one type of HSV (by either HSV 1 IgG or HSV 2 IgG) and positive HSV PCR isolation of another type
- Symptoms are milder due to partial protection

Recurrent infection

- This is defined as HSV infection in a woman who already has antibodies to that HSV type
- It occurs more frequently during the first three months after the primary infection
- There may be a few relatively painless vesicles that last for about a week

Diagnosis

- The majority of women with genital HSV infections (primary, non-primary and recurrent) are asymptomatic and unrecognised
- Routine screening for genital herpes with serology is at present not recommended
- Clinical diagnosis may be confirmed by type specific serology and viral culture
  - in asymptomatic women swab the cervix and the site of recurrence, even if no lesion is visualized
  - the culture report may take up to 7 days
  - a PCR can distinguish HSV 1 from HSV 2
    - results are usually available in 1-2 days
    - PCR testing has a potential for a higher detection rate than HSV culture

Perinatal transmission

- Most mothers of infants with neonatal HSV disease were previously unaware of their own infection
- Intrauterine infection may result in:
  - microcephaly
  - microphthalmia

    - intracranial calcifications
    - chorioretinitis
- Maternal HSV infection at the time of vaginal birth may lead to severe neonatal disease from ascending infection after the rupture of membranes
- Use of fetal-scalp electrode and fetal blood sampling increases the risk

Risk rates of transmission to fetus are:
- with primary infection, 50%
- with asymptomatic primary infection, 33%
- recurrent disease with active lesion, 2-3%
- recurrent disease that is asymptomatic, < 1%

Neonatal herpes
- Both HSV 1 and HSV 2 can cause neonatal herpes
- Most are acquired during vaginal birth
- Risk is highest with primary infection in the third trimester
- Clinically it can present as
    - localised infection on skin, eyes or mouth
    - encephalitis alone
        - it can develop 2-4 weeks after birth
    - disseminated herpes-multiorgan involvement

Management
- Ask all pregnant women at the first visit if they have a history of genital herpes
- At the onset of labour, again ask about symptoms of genital herpes
- Examine carefully for herpetic lesions
- Consult the neonatal team as needed

Primary infection in the first and second trimesters
- Recommend saline baths and topical anaesthetic agents
- Recommend Acyclovir (400mg orally three times daily for 5 days or Valacyclovir 500mg twice daily for 5 days) and analgesia as required
    - recommend commencing medication within 5 days of the onset of infection
- Recommend suppressive therapy as below for the remainder of the pregnancy or from 36 weeks to delivery
- Delivery
    - recommend vaginal birth if she has no active lesions when she arrives in labour

Primary infection in the third trimester

- Treat with Acyclovir as above to treat acute attack and for suppression
- Recommend elective CS at term
    - particularly if the symptoms occur within 6 weeks of expected delivery
    - the risk of neonatal transmission of HSV is very high with a vaginal birth

All women with active lesions on arrival in labour

- Recommend CS
- There may also be some benefit in performing CS beyond 4 hours of rupture of the membranes even though generally we allow a vaginal birth if the membranes have been ruptured for > 6 hours
    - the risk of transmission with a vaginal birth is 25-50%
- If a vaginal delivery is unavoidable or if the woman elects for a vaginal birth after a primary infection
    - avoid invasive procedures such as fetal scalp electrode monitoring and fetal blood sampling
    - if there is an obstetric indication to expedite delivery in the second stage, an operative delivery (instrumental or vacuum extraction) may be the safest mode; however, there is a small risk of transmission of HSV to the baby
    - recommend intrapartum intravenous Acyclovir 5mg/kg 8 hourly till birth to the mother and subsequently to the newborn to reduce neonatal herpes
    - notify the paediatrician and discuss swabs required at delivery

Women with genital herpes who present with PPROM

- Recommend immediate delivery by CS if term
- Recommend expectant management if preterm:
    - recommend intravenous Acyclovir 5 mg/kg every 8 hours for 24 to 48 hours and then orally
    - recommend prophylactic corticosteroids as normal
    - if delivery is indicated within 6 weeks of the primary infection, delivery by caesarean section may still offer some benefit despite the prolonged rupture of membranes

Recurrent genital herpes

- Antenatal swabbing is of no help
- Recommend suppressive therapy from 36 weeks of gestation or in some cases from the onset of first recurrence:
    - Acyclovir 400mg three times daily
    - Valacyclovir 500mg twice daily
- If there are active lesions or if she has any symptoms on arrival in labour
    - offer an elective CS
    - some would offer vaginal birth as risk of transmission is < 3%
    - risk of transmission is about 15% with HSV 1 and < 1% with HSV 2
- Offer a vaginal birth if membranes have been ruptured for > 6 hours
    - recommend Syntocinon infusion as soon as she arrives with spontaneous rupture of membranes without contracting
- Offer vaginal birth if no lesions are present

Neonatal management

- Asymptomatic infant with low risk of neonatal HSV disease (mother with recurrent genital infection, or primary genital or systemic infection that has seroconverted well prior to delivery with or without genital lesions at delivery)
    - recommend follow-up for clinical disease or testing for HSV PCR
- Asymptomatic infant with high risk of neonatal HSV disease (mother with primary genital or systemic infection close to delivery or infant born through birth canal with active HSV disease to mother with no prior history of genital herpes simplex infection)
    - test CSF for HSV PCR, blood count (for low platelets), LFTs, HSV PCR in blood
        - treat these neonates and those in the low risk group who develop a clinical disease
            - slow (1-2 hours) intravenous infusion of Acyclovir, 20mg/kg 3 times daily for 10-14 days
            - treat for 21 days if the neonate develops encephalitis or a disseminated disease

Recommended Reading

1. Money DM. No. 208 – Guidelines for the Management of Herpes Simplex Virus in Pregnancy. *J. Obstet. Gynaecol. Can.* 2017.
2. Palasanthiran P, Starr M, Jones C, Giles M, editors. *Management of perinatal infections.* Sydney: Australasian Society for Infectious Diseases (ASID) 2014. Available from: URL: http://www.asid.net.au/resources/clinical-guidelines
3. Royal College of Obstetricians and Gynaecologists (RCOG). Management of genital herpes in pregnancy. October 2014. Available from URL: https://www.rcog.org.uk
4. American College of Obstetricians and Gynecologists' Committee on Practice Bulletins—Obstetrics. ACOG Practice Bulletin. Management of Genital Herpes in Pregnancy - Number 220. *Obstet and Gynecol.* 2020 May; 135(5): e193-e202. doi: 0.1097/AOG.0000000000003840.
5. Sénat MV, Anselem O, Picone O et al. Prevention and management of genital herpes simplex infection during pregnancy and delivery: Guidelines from the French College of Gynaecologists and Obstetricians (CNGOF). *Eur. J. Obstet. Gynecol. Reprod. Biol.* 2018 May; 224:93-101. doi: 10.1016/j.ejogrb.2018.03.011.

CHAPTER TWENTY-NINE

HIV INFECTION IN PREGNANCY

- Offer HIV screening early in the pregnancy
- Consider third-trimester re-testing for Syphilis and HIV infection
- Discuss partner notification with women who have been recently diagnosed with HIV infection
- Diagnosing HIV and initiating antiretroviral therapy (ART) at the time of diagnosis are crucial to reducing the risk of perinatal HIV transmission and maintaining the health of pregnant women
- Manage the woman in a multidisciplinary team setting – HIV physician, specialist obstetrician, infectious disease consultant, infection control coordinator, neonatologist / paediatrician, anaesthetist, midwife and allied health services as appropriate

Investigations
- Full blood count, CD4 cell count and lymphocyte subsets
- HIV viral load
- Baseline bloods
    - liver function tests, electrolytes, urea, creatinine, amylase, lactate, and HLA B5701
    - swabs and urine screening
    - consider a low vaginal swab for genital and other sexually transmitted infections (Gonorrhoea, Chlamydia and Bacterial Vaginosis) and first void urine for Chlamydia

Antenatal Management
- Initiate ART early and suppress viral load during pregnancy and in labour

Rates of transmission are increased if:
- Advanced maternal illness is present
- The woman has a high maternal viral load (due to advanced infection or viral activity)

- The maternal status:
    - a low CD4 count
    - rupture of membranes > 4 hours before birth
    - a preterm birth
    - procedures that may jeopardise the integrity of natural barriers
        - fetal scalp electrodes
        - fetal blood sampling
        - vigorous suctioning
        - injections through unwashed skin
    - breast feeding

Mode of birth
Viral load < 50 copies/mL (undetectable) or CD4 ≥ 350 at or after 36 weeks gestation

- Continue current treatment
- There is no need for intrapartum ART
- Aim for a vaginal birth if there are no obstetric contraindications

Viral load 50-399 copies/mL at or after 36 weeks gestation

- Recommend intrapartum zidovudine
- Recommend elective CS between 38 and 39 weeks gestation

Viral load more than 400 copies/mL at or after 36 weeks gestation

- Recommend intrapartum zidovudine (see table below)
- Recommend a planned elective CS between 38 and 39 weeks gestation

If she is planning a caesarean section and presents with spontaneous rupture of the membranes (SROM) near term – offer a vaginal birth

- Aim to avoid prolonged labour
    - there is little data to support CS in this setting
- Consider use of forceps rather than a vacuum
    - forceps are less likely to damage the integrity of the skin

If she presents
with SROM between 34-37 weeks - recommend immediate delivery

- Recommend she doesn't breast feed
- Recommend lactation suppression with Cabergoline
- Continue ART in consultation with an infectious diseases consultant
- Discuss contraception

Recommended Reading

1. Pitts CJ. Update on Clinical Practice Guidelines for Human Immunodeficiency Virus. *Nurs. Clin. North Am.* 2020 Sep; 55(3): 417-427.
2. Gilleece DY, Tariq DS, Bamford DA et al. British HIV Association guidelines for the management of HIV in pregnancy and postpartum 2018. *HIV Med.* 2019 Mar; 20 Suppl 3: s2-s85.
3. Committee on Obstetric Practice; HIV Expert Work Group. ACOG Committee Opinion No. 751: Labor and Delivery Management of Women With Human Immunodeficiency Virus Infection. *Obstet Gynecol.* 2018 Sep; 132(3): e131-e137.
4. Bailey H, Zash R, Rasi V, Thorne C. HIV treatment in pregnancy. *Lancet HIV*. 2018 Aug; 5(8): e457-e467.
5. Zar FA. Guideline: Recommendations are provided for antiretroviral therapies in pregnant women with HIV. *Ann. Intern. Med.* 2018; 168(4).
6. Loutfy M, Kennedy VL, Poliquin V et al. No. 354-Canadian HIV Pregnancy Planning Guidelines. *J. Obstet. Gynaecol. Can.* 2018 Jan; 40(1): 94-114.

CHAPTER THIRTY

HYPERTENSION IN PREGNANCY

Incidence: 10-15% of all pregnancies – pre-eclampsia occurs in 3-5% of pregnancies.

Normal changes in pregnancy

- There is a fall in blood pressure (BP) during the first and second trimesters and then a rise in the third trimester

Definitions of hypertension (HT) include

- Systolic BP $\geq$ 140mm Hg or diastolic BP $\geq$ 90mm Hg on at least 2 readings measured 5-10 minutes apart and ideally over several hours
- a single reading of systolic BP $\geq$ 170mm Hg or diastolic BP $\geq$ 110mm Hg
    - mild - diastolic BP 90–99mm Hg, systolic BP 140–149mm Hg
    - moderate - diastolic BP 100–109mm Hg, systolic BP 150–159mm Hg.
    - severe - diastolic BP 110mm Hg or greater, systolic BP 170mm Hg or greater
- a rise of > 30mm Hg systolic BP or > 15mm Hg diastolic BP has also been used

Prevention of hypertension in pregnancy - mostly pre-eclampsia (PE)

- Recommend lifestyle changes: weight control with healthy eating and physical exercise
- Recommend low dose of Aspirin (150mg at bedtime) and calcium (600mg twice daily) from 7 weeks gestation. It can however start at any time up to 16 weeks and continue till 36 weeks, to prevent PE, in women with:
    - a history of PE in previous pregnancy
    - chronic renal disease
    - an autoimmune disease including antiphospholipid syndrome
    - type 1 and 2 diabetes
    - chronic hypertension

  - if more than one of the following applies:
    - first pregnancy
    - age ≥ 40 years
    - BMI ≥ 35kg/m^2
    - pregnancy interval > 10 years
    - family history of pre-eclampsia
    - multiple pregnancy
- There may be some role also for the use of Metformin
- Currently data do not support use of heparin for prevention of pre-eclampsia
- Newer options may include use of Statins

Assessment of proteinuria

- Recommend using an automated reagent-strip reading device or a spot urinary protein-creatinine ratio (PCR) for estimating proteinuria
- There is no advantage in doing a 24-hour collection for proteinuria
- There is no benefit in repeating PCR once it is elevated (> 30 mg/mmol)

Classification

1. Chronic hypertension

- This refers to the woman being known to be hypertensive prior to pregnancy or having been diagnosed with hypertension before 20 weeks gestation
- If diagnosed with hypertension for the first time:
  - look for a possible cause for the hypertension
    - essential hypertension
    - secondary hypertension
      - renal – chronic nephritis, polycystic kidneys, rental artery stenosis
      - cardiac – coarctation of aorta
      - endocrine – Cushing's, Conns, Phaeochromocytoma and rarely hyperparathyroidism
      - systemic diseases with renal involvement – diabetes and systemic lupus erythematosus (SLE)
    - white coat hypertension

- Risks to woman with chronic HT include:
    - accelerated HT in the third trimester
    - superimposed pre-eclampsia (25% risk)
    - fetal growth restriction
    - placental abruption
    - preterm birth (28%)
    - stillbirth

Management is usually done in conjunction with a physician

- Recommend screening for secondary causes of hypertension
    - examine femoral pulses, listen for renal bruit, and perform urine and other blood tests
- Control blood pressure
    - aim to keep blood pressure 120-130/80-85 (strict control of BP to low normal values appears to be advantageous)
    - if she is on ACE inhibitors advise stopping them and recommend changing to an alternative medication
    - bed rest is of no benefit and may even be harmful (recommend reducing physical activity)
    - use appropriate hypotensive drugs
        - first line – Methyl Dopa 250-750mg three times daily
            - it may cause dry mouth, depression, drowsiness, postural hypotension
        - Labetalol 100-400mg three times daily in addition to the above if required
            - it can cause headaches
        - Nifedipine – 20mg twice daily
        - Prazosin – 0.5-5mg three times daily
        - Hydralazine - 25-50mg three times daily
    - if she develops acute severe HT (systolic $\geq$ 170 or diastolic $\geq$ 110), recommend:
        - Nifedipine – 20mg orally and repeat in 30 minutes if required
        - Labetalol – 20mg intravenously over 2 minutes and repeat after 10 minutes if required
        - Hydralazine – 5-10mg intravenously and repeat after another 20 minutes if required
- Monitor for signs of superimposed pre-eclampsia
    - assess for proteinuria at every visit
    - request pre-eclampsia bloods (see list below)

- Monitor for and manage any maternal complications especially if the hypertension is worsening
    - o urine for protein (a spot urine protein/creatinine ratio)
    - o urine microscopy (red cells and casts)
    - o serum electrolytes, liver function tests including LDH, creatinine and urates
    - o full blood count
- Monitor fetal growth and wellbeing (see chapter on fetal growth and wellbeing)
- Plan birth
    - o if blood pressure is well controlled and there are no complications, await spontaneous labour or offer induction of labour at around 40 weeks
    - o if there is any concern with blood pressure or fetal growth – consider birth after 37 weeks
- Postpartum – blood pressure is usually unstable for 1-2 weeks after delivery especially on days 3-6 and may be difficult to control
    - o maintain current hypotensive medication for 24 hours
    - o then consider going back on previous medication prior to pregnancy or commence ACE inhibitors such as Captopril
    - o avoid Methyl Dopa (risk of postpartum depression)
- Ensure she has a follow up appointment with her General Practitioner

2. Gestational hypertension

- High BP is detected for the first time in the second half of the pregnancy; BP is usually mildly elevated
    - o usually there is no proteinuria
    - o some women diagnosed with gestational HT may in fact be in the early process of developing PE
    - o consider PE in a primigravida who develops "gestational hypertension" near term
    - o gestational hypertension usually resolves within 3 months of birth
- It is usually associated with good prognosis
- She has a higher risk of developing chronic hypertension later in life

Manage like with chronic hypertension

- o control blood pressure
- o monitor for complications or development of pre-eclampsia
- o monitor maternal and fetal wellbeing

  - plan delivery
    - if diastolic < 100 and no complications – await spontaneous labour or induction at around 40 weeks
    - if diastolic ≥ 100 or there are any concerns, consider delivery from 37 weeks
- Postpartum
  - maintain current hypotensive medication for 24 hours and then consider ACE inhibitors such as Captopril until BP returns to normal
  - avoid Methyl Dopa as its use may increase risk of postpartum depression
  - ensure she has a follow up appointment with her General Practitioner
  - later in life she is at:
    - higher risk of developing chronic HT
    - higher risk of recurrence
      - advise on lifestyle change – weight and exercise

3. Pre-eclampsia

- Hypertension is detected for the first time after 20 weeks gestation and associated with other criteria mentioned below
- This is a multiorgan disorder of unknown aetiology
- Although proteinuria is most commonly present, it is not mandatory to make the diagnosis

Risk factors for Pre-eclampsia:

- General
  - age > 40 years or < 20 years
  - BMI > 30kg/m^2
- Genetic
  - PE in the mother (1 in 4 will get it) and if a sister had it (1 in 3 may get it)
- Obstetric factors
  - nulliparity
  - past history of PE
    - 1% if they've never had it
    - 5-7% if they've had uncomplicated PE
    - 60% if they've had early onset severe PE
  - multiple pregnancy

- short sexual relationship before conception
- assisted reproduction
- interpregnancy interval > 5 years
- triploidy

- Medical factors
  - chronic hypertension
  - renal disease
  - diabetes
  - anti-phospholipid syndrome and connective tissue diseases
- "Pre-eclampsia" < 20 weeks may be associated with hydatidiform mole or Triploidy

Predicting development of PE

- There may be failure of BP to drop in the 2nd trimester
- An abnormal uterine artery doppler at 18-20 weeks increases the risk of developing pre-eclampsia and/or intrauterine growth restriction six-fold
  - it has however a high negative predictive value
- Angiogenic factors:
  - sFlt-1/PlGF ratio > 35 has been shown by some as an indicator of developing pre-eclampsia in the next 7 days
  - high sFlt levels
  - low levels of PlGF (< 0.3 MoM) have been shown to be independently associated with spontaneous preterm birth, pre-eclampsia and a composite adverse pregnancy outcome
    - it may have more of a role as a negative predictive value for pre-eclampsia

Diagnosis

- Preeclampsia is diagnosed when hypertension > 20 weeks occurs with one or more of the following (note proteinuria is no longer a prerequisite)
  - renal involvement
    - significant proteinuria – spot urine protein/creatinine ratio ≥ 30mg/mmol
    - serum or plasma creatinine > 90µmol/l
    - oliguria
  - haematological involvement
    - thrombocytopenia
    - haemolysis
    - disseminated intravascular coagulation

  - liver involvement
    - raised serum transaminases
      - severe epigastric or right upper quadrant pain that responds poorly to analgesia
  - neurological involvement
    - convulsions (eclampsia)
    - hyperreflexia with sustained clonus
    - severe headache
    - persistent visual disturbances (flashing before eyes, blurring or loss of vision)
  - pulmonary oedema – a rare feature of acute left ventricular failure
  - fetal growth restriction
  - placental abruption
- Beware of oedema of the face and fingers
- Raised uric acid is not a diagnostic feature of PE
  - in early pregnancy (≤ 32 weeks) a high or rising level correlates with poor fetal prognosis – rising levels over a few days would be concerning

HELLP Syndrome is a manifestation of severe PE
- Diagnosis requires at least 2 of the following:
  - haemolysis
    - abnormal peripheral blood film with burr cells
    - elevated bilirubin ≥ 1.2mg/dl
    - increased LDH > twice the upper limit of what is normal
  - elevated liver enzymes ≥ twice the upper limit of what is normal
  - low platelet < 100000
    - risk of spontaneous bleeding is not significantly increased until the count falls below 50000
    - consider ultrasound or CT scan of the liver to exclude liver haematoma

Management of pre-eclampsia – usually working with the physician
- Control hypertension
- Monitor for severity of pre-eclampsia
  - mild: BP 140-149/90-99 and /or proteinuria – nil - +
  - mod: BP 150-159/100-109 and/or proteinuria + - ++

  - severe: BP 170 or above/110 or above and/or proteinuria +++ or above
  - imminent eclampsia: with clinical features of CNS irritability
- Monitor for feto-maternal complications (tests as for chronic hypertension above)
- Monitor fetal growth and wellbeing (see section on fetal growth and wellbeing)
- Prevent convulsions
- Plan delivery – delivery is the only cure for pre-eclampsia
  - indications for delivery include:
    - hypertension and raised PCR at gestation of 37 weeks or more
    - placental abruption
    - inability to control blood pressure despite treatment
    - falling platelet levels – a count < 100,000
    - deteriorating liver enzymes
    - deteriorating renal function – serum creatinine
    - coagulopathy
    - concern regarding fetal welfare – fetal distress, severe FGR, or abnormal dopplers
    - eclampsia
    - placental growth factor and the sFlt-1/PlGF ratio show promise for prognosticating adverse outcomes in preeclampsia, but study heterogeneity limits their clinical utility
- Aim for a vaginal birth
  - inform the anaesthetist
  - monitor and control blood pressure ½ hourly
  - observe urine output 4 hourly
  - ensure she has continuous fetal heart rate monitoring
  - analgesia
    - obtain early anaesthetist consultation
    - epidural analgesia controls blood pressure and prevents BP fluctuations
  - ensure satisfactory coagulation tests and platelet count
  - assist the second stage if blood pressure is high or labile
  - actively manage the third stage – do not use ergometrine

Other considerations

- Fluid control – avoid fluid overload as she may develop pulmonary oedema

  - oliguria is common early postpartum and does not require fluid therapy unless the serum plasma creatinine is rising
  - ensure strict fluid balance monitoring
  - restrict post-birth intravenous crystalloids to 1500mL in the first 24 hours
  - persistent oliguria beyond 24 hours postpartum with rising plasma creatinine suggests the possibility of postpartum renal failure
- Recommend Magnesium Sulphate if:
  - she has hyperreflexia (sustained clonus)
  - she has evidence of cerebral irritability
  - HELLP syndrome
    - 4g loading dose over 5 min and then 1g/hour
- Recommend platelet transfusion – if < 50000
- Recommend thromboprophylaxis – TEDs stockings and Clexane if she's an inpatient (see chapter on thromboembolism)

Postpartum care

- Eclampsia may occur postpartum
- Postpartum hypertension is common – it may only peak on days 3-6 if not previously hypertensive
  - if the woman is on Labetalol – stop within 24-48 hours and change over to Captopril
  - advise to continue this for 2 weeks with a GP follow up
  - avoid Methyl Dopa as noted above
- If on Magnesium Sulphate, continue for 24 hours after delivery
- Oliguria - oliguria is common especially after induction of labour or operative birth
  - avoid aggressive fluid therapy as it may cause pulmonary oedema
  - avoid diuretics unless clinically indicated for fluid overload
- Mortality – the commonest cause of death is cerebral haemorrhage. Other causes include multiorgan failure and adult respiratory distress syndrome

Resolution of pre-eclampsia

- During the first 1-2 days after delivery, liver enzyme elevations and thrombocytopenia often deteriorate
- Hypertension may persist for days and even up to three months
- Advise about risk of recurrence in future pregnancies

4. Chronic Hypertension with superimposed preeclampsia

- One or more of the systemic features of pre-eclampsia may develop after 20 weeks of gestation in a woman with chronic hypertension

5. Eclampsia

- Seizures occur in women who have had pre-eclampsia
- Only 1 in 3 women would have had a diagnosis of PE in the previous week
    - 40% of attacks are antepartum, 20% are intrapartum and 40% are postpartum
- Teenagers are 3 times more at risk for eclampsia than older women
- It is more common in nulliparous women (20% are in multiparous women with no previous history of pre-eclampsia)
- Cortical blindness is usually transient from vasospasm of the retinal artery – it may also be due to retinal detachment
- Aims of management include:
    - resuscitation
    - controlling blood pressure
    - controlling seizures – use magnesium sulphate as above
    - if they cannot be controlled or recur, recommend using
        - Diazepam 5–10mg IV at a rate of 2–5 mg/minute (maximum dose of 10mg)
        - Midazolam 5–10mg IV over 2–5 minutes
        - Clonazepam 1–2mg IV over 2–5 minutes
    - assess fetal well being
    - assess for coagulopathy
    - stabilise the woman before rushing for delivery
        - correct coagulopathy
        - control blood pressure

Recommended Reading

1. SOMANZ – The SOMANZ Guidelines for the management of hypertensive disorders of pregnancy 2014.
2. Nirupama R, Divyashree S, Janhavi P et al. Preeclampsia: Pathophysiology and Management. *J. Gynecol. Obstet. Hum. Reprod.*, 2020 Nov 7.
3. Whitney A Booker Hypertensive Disorders of Pregnancy, *Clin. Perinatol.* 2020 Dec; 47(4): 817-833.

4. Suksai M, Geater A, Phumsiripaiboon P, Suntharasaj T. A new risk score model to predict preeclampsia using maternal factors and mean arterial pressure in early pregnancy. *J. Obstet. Gynaecol.* 2021 Jun 21: 1-6.
5. Gebremedhin AT, Tessema GA, Regan AK, Pereira G. Association between interpregnancy interval and hypertensive disorders of pregnancy: Effect modification by maternal age. *Paediatr. Perinat. Epidemiol.* 2021 Jul; 35(4): 415-424.
6. Zhang Y, Liang C, Wang C et al. Lower blood pressure achieved leads to better pregnant outcomes in non-severe chronic hypertensive pregnant women. *Pregnancy Hypertens.* 2021 May 14; 25: 62-67.
7. Chappell LC, Cluver CA, Kingdom J, Tong S. Pre-eclampsia. *Lancet.* 2021 May 27: S0140-6736(20)32335-7. doi: 10.1016/S0140-6736(20)32335-7.
8. Ekelund CK, Rode L, Tabor A et al. Placental Growth Factor and Adverse Obstetric Outcomes in a Mixed-Risk Cohort of Women Screened for Preeclampsia in the First Trimester of Pregnancy. *Fetal Diagn. Ther.* 2021; 48(4): 304-312.
9. Duhig KE, Seed PT, Placzek A et al. Prognostic indicators of severe disease in late preterm pre-eclampsia to guide decision making on timing of delivery: The PEACOCK study. *Pregnancy Hypertens.* 2021 Jun; 24: 90-95.
10. Lim S, Li W, Kemper J et al. Biomarkers and the Prediction of Adverse Outcomes in Preeclampsia: A Systematic Review and Meta-analysis. *Obstet. Gynecol.* 2021 Jan 1; 137(1): 72-81.
11. Hodel M, Blank PR, Marty P, Lapaire O. sFlt-1/PlGF Ratio as a Predictive Marker in Women with Suspected Preeclampsia: An Economic Evaluation from a Swiss Perspective. *Dis. Markers.* 2019 Aug 14; 2019: 4096847. doi: 10.1155/2019/4096847.
12. Cerdeira AS, O'Sullivan J, Ohuma EO et al. Randomized Interventional Study on Prediction of Preeclampsia/Eclampsia in Women With Suspected Preeclampsia: INSPIRE. *Hypertension.* 2019 Oct; 74(4): 983-990.

CHAPTER THIRTY-ONE

HYPERTHYROIDISM IN PREGNANCY

- Normal values of TSH in pregnancy are trimester dependent:
    - first trimester – 0.1- 2.5mIU/L
    - second trimester – 0.2–3.0mIU/L
    - third trimester – 0.3–3.0mIU/L
- 0.1-0.4% in pregnancy
    - Graves' disease is responsible for 95% of cases
        - it is an autoimmune disorder caused by thyroid stimulating hormone (TSH) receptor antibodies
    - others include
        - transient gestational hyperthyroidism
        - toxic adenoma
        - multinodular goitre
        - gestational trophoblastic tumours
    - currently routine screening for thyroid dysfunction is not recommended – test high risk cases:
        - history of thyroid dysfunction or surgery
        - recurrent miscarriages
        - family history of thyroid disease
        - type 1 diabetes
        - presence of goitre
        - history of autoimmune disorder, high-dose neck radiation or postpartum thyroid dysfunction
        - previous delivery of infant with thyroid disease
        - morbid obesity

Preconception counselling

- Emphasise the importance of achieving and maintaining euthyroid function before conception

Clinical features

- Women usually do not present for the first time in pregnancy – most cases are already known

  - if it does occur, it usually presents in late first or early second trimester
- Features mimic changes of normal pregnancy
- Activity may fluctuate in pregnancy – may exacerbate in the first trimester and postpartum with gradual remission in the second half of the pregnancy
  - weight loss, persistent tachycardia, palpitations, and tremor are consistent features

Diagnosis

- Low serum TSH levels (often < 0.01mU/l)
- Raised serum free T4 or T3 levels
- In early pregnancy, test for thyroid receptor antibodies (TRab) – these include thyroid stimulating immunoglobulin (TSI) and TSH binding inhibitory immunoglobulin

Effect of pregnancy on hyperthyroidism

- It often improves
- The woman may need lower doses of treatment as their pregnancy advances

Effect of untreated hyperthyroidism on pregnancy

- **Fetal**
  - miscarriage
  - congenital malformations
  - fetal growth restriction
  - stillbirth
  - fetal and neonatal thyrotoxicosis.
- **Maternal**
  - maternal sinus tachycardia and supraventricular tachycardia
  - retrosternal goitre – may cause tracheal obstruction
  - placental abruption
  - preeclampsia
  - preterm labour
  - thyroid storm (if poorly controlled, especially during labour)

Management – to be carried out in conjunction with physicians

Ensure she is euthyroid as soon as possible

- Monitor fetal growth

- Recommend an ultrasound of the maternal thyroid
- If she is smoking, advise her to stop as it can exacerbate eye changes
- Seek anaesthetic opinion
- Medication
    - Thioamides - Carbimazole or Propylthiouracil (PTU) – both can cause agranulocytosis – so be watchful
        - if planning a pregnancy or diagnosed for the first time in pregnancy – recommend Propylthiouracil (PTU) in the first trimester as Carbimazole is associated with a rare embryopathy
            - start with 100-150 mg three times daily and reduce to 50mg 1-2 times daily once controlled
        - Carbimazole – change to Carbimazole after first trimester as PTU can cause fulminant hepatitis
            - the usual dose is 10-15mg three times daily
    - beta-blockers – Propranolol 10-40mg three times daily to control severe symptoms or until antithyroid medication works
- Monitor serum TSH – maintain TSH and keep T4 levels at around or slightly above upper normal using the lowest drug dose
- Monitor TRab every trimester and TFT every 4 weeks

Surgical treatment

- Surgery is necessary if goitre is causing tracheal compression
    - surgery in pregnancy is only performed as a last resort
    - if required, perform during the latter part of the second trimester

Fetal/neonatal thyrotoxicosis

- This can occur especially if the disease is active in the third trimester
- TRab cross the placenta and increase the risk of fetal and neonatal hyperthyroidism, diagnosed by noting:
    - persistent fetal tachycardia
    - excessive fetal movements after about 34 weeks

    - in all women who are TRab positive, arrange an ultrasound scan of the fetus, screening for FGR, fetal goitre, fused skull bones, hydrops, oligo or polyhydramnios
- If TRab levels are significantly high (> 3 times upper limit of normal), recommend:
    - an ultrasound scan of the fetal thyroid at 24-28 weeks
    - a weekly CTG to detect persistent fetal tachycardia
    - that the woman report any feeling of excessive fetal movements

Labour and delivery

- Aim for spontaneous labour at term – monitor maternal pulse and FHR to diagnose thyroid storm
- Cord blood can also be tested for fetal thyroid status

Neonatal hyperthyroidism

- Recommend paediatric review at 6 hours of birth
- Condition may be delayed for a day to a week while maternal drug treatment is cleared
- Usually self-limiting to about 3 months
- Weight loss, poor weight gain, tachycardia and irritability are early signs

Breast feeding

- It is safe to breast feed – moderate doses of antithyroid drugs appear to be safe
    - as far as is practical, advise women to take medication after the baby has been breastfed

Recommended Reading

1. Leo A et al. Thyroid disease in pregnancy. *Amer. Fam. Physician* 2014; 89(4): 273-9.
2. Thyroid Disease in Pregnancy: ACOG Practice Bulletin, Number 223. American College of Obstetricians and Gynecologists' Committee on Practice Bulletins—Obstetrics. *Obstet. Gynecol.* 2020 Jun; 135(6): e261-e274.
3. Kahaly GJ. Management of Graves Thyroidal and Extrathyroidal Disease: An Update. *J. Clin. Endocrinol Metab.* 2020 Dec 1; 105(12): dgaa646.

4. Zhou M, Wang M, Li J, Luo X, Lei M. Effects of thyroid diseases on pregnancy outcomes. *Exp. Ther. Med.* 2019 Sep; 18(3): 1807-1815.

CHAPTER THIRTY-TWO

HYPOTHYROIDISM IN PREGNANCY

- Occurs in 1-2% of pregnancies – the majority are subclinical
- Normal values of TSH in pregnancy are trimester dependent:
    - first trimester – 0.1- 2.5 mIU/L
    - second trimester – 0.2–3.0mIU/L
    - third trimester – 0.3–3.0mIU/L

1. Subclinical hypothyroidism – normal fT3 and fT4

- If TSH is < 2.5mIU/l
    - no further treatment is required
- If TSH is 2.5-4.0
    - test for anti-thyroid antibodies (thyroid peroxidase antibody [TPO ab]) and thyroid anti-globulin antibodies)
        - if positive
            - commence thyroxine 50mcg/day
        - if negative
            - no further treatment is required
- If TSH is > 4.0
    - recommend thyroxine 50mcg daily
- With all women, repeat TSH measurement in 4 weeks
    - if TSH is above the recommended level increase thyroxine to 75mcg daily
    - if TSH is < 0.4mIU/l reduce dose to 25mcg daily
        - then repeat TSH at 18, 26 and 34 weeks
            - aim for TSH values within the trimester specific reference range

Postpartum

- Cease thyroxine and retest 4-6 weeks postpartum

2. Clinical hypothyroidism – high TSH and low fT3 and fT_4 levels

Screening

- Currently routine screening for thyroid dysfunction is not recommended – test high risk cases:
  - history of thyroid dysfunction or thyroid surgery
  - recurrent miscarriages
  - family history of thyroid disease
  - type 1 diabetes
  - goitre
  - history of autoimmune disorder, high-dose neck radiation or postpartum thyroid dysfunction
  - previous delivery of infant with thyroid disease
  - morbid obesity

Aetiology

- Chronic autoimmune thyroiditis (Hashimoto's disease) is the commonest cause and is associated with antithyroid peroxidase antibodies
- Previously treated Graves' disease
- Surgery to thyroid
- Iodine deficiency

Preconception counselling:

- Provide advice on the importance of achieving normal thyroid function before conception
- There is a need for immediate monitoring at the onset of pregnancy, because by the first antenatal visit, many women will already have an elevated TSH level consistent with uncontrolled hypothyroidism
- Advise women who are well controlled to increase their medication by two additional doses per week after a missed menstrual cycle

Clinical features:

- Common symptoms include lack of energy and tiredness, weight gain, decreased exercise capacity, and constipation
- Other symptoms include hair loss, dry skin, constipation, mental disturbance, bradycardia and myotonic (slow relaxing) reflexes
- Some people will have cold intolerance, slow pulse rate and a delayed relaxation of tendon reflexes

Effect of hypothyroidism on pregnancy:

- Associated with subfertility
- If it is untreated or poorly controlled there is an increased risk of:
    - anaemia
    - gestational hypertension and pre-eclampsia
    - placental abruption
    - preterm labour and low birth weight
    - fetal neurocognitive deficits
    - stillbirth
        - treatment reduces risk of miscarriage, preterm birth and fetal intellectual development; however, it has little effect on risk of hypertension and placental abruption

Effect of pregnancy on hypothyroidism

- Often it is necessary to increase thyroid medication doses

Management

- If there is a palpable goitre, exclude retrosternal extension
- As hypothyroidism may coexist with Insulin dependent diabetes – request TFT when booking in women with pre-existing diabetes
- TPO antibodies – in Hashimoto's thyroiditis, thyroid peroxidase antibodies are present in 90% of cases and these cross the placenta; a level of > 50iu/ml increases the risk of placental abruption
- Recommend Thyroxine 100-200mcg once daily
    - advise the woman to take it on an empty stomach
    - assess thyroid function once in each trimester – keep TSH levels ≤ 2.5mIU/l
    - if taking iron, advise they take it and the thyroid medication 4 hours apart

Postpartum

- Decrease Thyroxine to pre-pregnancy dosage over a four-week period
- It is safe to breast-feed

Recommended Reading

1. Leo A. Thyroid disease in pregnancy. *Amer. Fam. Physician* 2014; 89(4): 273-9.
2. Thyroid Disease in Pregnancy: ACOG Practice Bulletin, Number 223. American College of Obstetricians and Gynecologists' Committee on

Practice Bulletins—Obstetrics. *Obstet. Gynecol.* 2020 Jun; 135(6): e261-e274.

3. Wilson SA, Stem LA, Bruehlman RD. Hypothyroidism: Diagnosis and Treatment. *Am. Fam. Physician*. 2021 May 15; 103(10): 605-613.
4. Li P, Lin S, Cui J et al. Impact of Early Pregnancy Subclinical Hypothyroidism on Gestational Diabetes Mellitus: A Retrospective Study of 7,536 Cases. *J. Women's Health* (Larchmt). 2021 Apr 7. doi: 10.1089/jwh.2020.8825.
5. Lee SY, Pearce EN. Testing, Monitoring, and Treatment of Thyroid Dysfunction in Pregnancy. *J. Clin. Endocrinol. Metab.* 2021 Mar 8; 106(3): 883-892.
6. Andersen SL, Andersen S. Turning to Thyroid Disease in Pregnant Women. *Eur. Thyroid J.* 2020 Sep; 9(5): 225-233.

CHAPTER THIRTY-THREE

IDIOPATHIC INTRACRANIAL HYPERTENSION

It is also called benign intracranial hypertension.

- It is more common in women and more so in women with high BMI
  - it may present for the first time in pregnancy
    - when that happens, it's often in the second trimester

Clinical features

- These include nausea, vomiting and headache (often retro orbital) and may cause visual impairment (double vision)
- There may be rapid weight gain
  - it may get worse during pregnancy and improve after birth

Diagnosis

- Diagnosis is made by exclusion
- There is papilloedema
- Intracranial pressure is raised with:
  - normal CT head (if done prior to pregnancy)
    - no hydrocephalus
    - no space occupying lesion
  - normal MRI during pregnancy

Management

- Liaise with physician and/or neurologist
- Advise the woman to avoid too much weight gain
- Treat persistent headaches
- Aim to reduce intracranial pressure
  - Acetazolamide is the preferred option
    - avoid it in the first trimester - if used in the first trimester advise a high dose of folic acid
    - its use in the third trimester can cause neonatal electrolyte imbalance
      - monitor electrolytes after birth

  - diuretics
  - steroids
  - repeated lumber punctures or a shunt
- Test visual acuity every 2 months during pregnancy
  - infarction of the optic nerve leading to blindness may occur
    - if there is deterioration use steroids promptly
- Refer to an anaesthetist in the third trimester

Labour
- If there is no deterioration await normal labour and birth
- Use analgesia in labour:
  - an epidural is ideal
  - avoid Pethidine and Morphine – reduction in pCO2 may cause an increase in cerebral blood flow and possibly raise CSF pressure
  - general anaesthesia may also increase CSF pressure.

Recurrence
- 10% in subsequent pregnancy

Recommended Reading

1. Bagga R, Jain V, Das CP et al. Choice of therapy and mode of delivery in idiopathic intracranial hypertension during pregnancy. *Med. Gen. Med.* 2005 Nov 10; 7(4): 42.
2. Tang RA. Management of idiopathic intracranial hypertension in pregnancy. *Med. Gen. Med.* 2005 Nov 10; 7(4): 40.
3. Alves S, Sousa N, Cardoso L et al. Multidisciplinary management of idiopathic intracranial hypertension in pregnancy: case series and narrative review. *Anesthesiol.* 2021 Mar 20: S0104-0014.
4. Park DSJ, Park JSY, Sharma S, Sharma RA. Idiopathic Intracranial Hypertension in Pregnancy. *J. Obstet. Gynaecol. Can.* 2021 Jan 4: S1701-2163.

CHAPTER THIRTY-FOUR

INDUCTION OF LABOUR

Induction of labour (IOL) is indicated when the maternal and/or fetal risks of ongoing pregnancy outweigh the risks of IOL.

Specific indications and their recommended gestational age for IOL

- Post dates
  - offer induction of labour at 41^0-41^6 weeks
- Advanced maternal age
  - nulliparous age over 35 years
    - offer induction between 40^0-40^6 weeks
  - nulliparous and multiparous age ≥ 40 years
    - offer induction at 39^0-39^6 weeks
- High BMI – no GDM or macrosomia
  - BMI > 40
    - offer induction of labour at 41^0-41^6 weeks
  - BMI > 50
    - offer CTG twice weekly at 38^0, 38^4 and 39^0 weeks because of the higher risk of perinatal death
    - offer induction of labour at 39^0-39^6 weeks
- Diabetes in pregnancy – no macrosomia
  - well controlled GDM on diet alone
    - offer IOL at 40^6-41^6 weeks as for post dates
  - well controlled GDM on metformin alone
    - offer IOL at 39^0-39^6 weeks
  - any GDM or type 2 diabetes on metformin AND insulin
    - offer IOL 38^0-38^6
  - type 1 diabetes on insulin
    - offer induction of labour at 38^0-38^6 weeks
  - well controlled type 2 diabetic or GDM on insulin
    - offer induction of labour at 38^0-38^6 weeks

- Multiple pregnancy
    - uncomplicated DCDA twins
        - offer induction of labour at 38^0 weeks
    - uncomplicated MCDA twins
        - offer induction of labour at 37^0 weeks
- Fetal growth restriction/SGA
    - if a constitutionally small fetus
        - continue to monitor it weekly
        - await spontaneous labour and induce at 40^0 weeks
    - if fetal growth restriction has occurred
        - for oligohydramnios – deliver by 37^0 weeks at the latest
        - if normal liquor volume – aim to get to and offer IOL at 38^0 -38^6 weeks if dopplers and CTG continue to remain normal
- Fetal macrosomia and no previous history of shoulder dystocia – with or without diabetes
    - EFW > 3500 at 36 weeks
    - EFW > 3700 at 37 weeks
    - EFW > 3900 at 38 weeks
        - offer induction as for diabetes at 38^0-38^6 weeks
- If the woman smokes (> 10 cigarettes per day)
    - offer a scan for growth at 37 weeks
    - offer IOL at 40^0 weeks if there are any concerns
- Obstetric cholestasis
    - note that women do not need to be fasting to monitor bile acid levels
    - regarding timing of birth:
        - if bile acid levels are < 40mmol/l deliver at 39-40 weeks
        - if they are 40-99mmol/l deliver at 38 weeks
        - if they are > 40mmol/l with deteriorating liver enzymes or severe symptoms despite being on UDCA advise delivery at 37^0-37^6 weeks
        - if they are ≥ 100 mmol/l deliver at 35-36 weeks
- Maternal request
    - generally we do not offer IOL on request where there is no medical or social indication
    - this is an individualised decision between the consultant and the woman

Preventing the need for IOL

Membrane sweep:

- Recommend membrane sweeps as they shorten the time to onset of spontaneous labour and reduce the need for formal induction for post dates
  - this may be performed every 2-3 days from 38 weeks
  - if the cervix is closed, a cervical massage in the vaginal fornices may achieve a similar effect
  - Group B Streptococcus (GBS) colonization does not contraindicate a membrane sweep

Assessment on admission for IOL

- Review of maternal history and check and confirm membranes are still intact
- Confirm gestation
- Check GBS status if available
- Palpate abdomen to measure fundal height and confirm presentation (preferably with a bed side scan)
- Assess fetal wellbeing with CTG (confirm it is normal)
- Assess Bishop score (BS)
  - cervical length is an important predictor of success or failure of IOL
  - the cervix is unfavourable if the score is 6 or less
  - a modified Bishop score is commonly used
  - a simplified Bishop score (as shown below) and adding parity have a better positive predictive value for a successful IOL

Modified Bishop Score

	0	1	2	3
Dilatation (cms)	< 1	1-2	3-4	> 4
Cervical length (cms)	≥ 3	2	1	< 1
Station	-3	-2	-1/0	+1/+2
Consistency	Firm	Medium	Soft	-
Position	Posterior	Mid	Anterior	-

Simplified scoring system

SCORE	0	1	2	3
Dilatation (cm)	< 1	1-2	3-4	> 4
Cervical length (cm)	> 3	2	1	< 1
Station	-3	-2	-1/0	≥ +1
Parity	0		≥ 1	

Methods for making the cervical score favourable – when the Bishop score is 6 or less

Double balloon catheter

- Use the double balloon catheter for:
    - all multiparous women
    - women with one previous caesarean section
    - all nulliparous women with a Bishop score (BS) of 4 or more
        - there is good evidence of safety for outpatient management until the first assessment at 12 hours post insertion
        - there is no need for CTG post insertion
        - if the catheter gets expelled
            - perform an amniotomy if the BS is 7 or more
        - if it does not get expelled – reassess at 12 and 18 hours post insertion
            - if then the catheter gets expelled or if the BS is 7 or more at either assessment
                - perform an amniotomy
            - if the BS is 6 or less
                - recommend Cervidil at 0600 and reassess at 1800 and 2400hrs
                    - perform an amniotomy if the BS > 6 at either assessment
                    - if the BS is still 4-6 perform an amniotomy if possible
                    - if the BS is still < 4 consider:
                        - an amniotomy

- postponing for 24 hours
- caesarean section (CS)

Prostaglandins
Cervidil

- Use Cervidil for
  - all nulliparous women with a BS of < 4
    - assess the BS at 18 and 24hrs post insertion
      - remove the pessary and perform an amniotomy if the BS is 7 or more
      - remove the pessary also if
        - her membranes rupture
        - she gets painful regular contractions for an hour
        - uterine hyperstimulation occurs – but ONLY IF she has > 5 painful contractions and there are FHR concerns
    - if the BS is still < 4 at 24 hours after insertion
      - insert a double balloon catheter and reassess 12 and 18 hours later
        - as soon as the catheter is expelled
          - perform an amniotomy if the BS is 7 or more
        - if the catheter does not fall out
          - perform an amniotomy if the BS is 7 or more at either assessment
          - if the cervical score is still < 4 consider:
            - an amniotomy
            - postponement
            - a CS

PG Gel

- Use PG gel in the same manner as for Cervidil
- It is associated with a lower incidence of hyperstimulation
  - all nulliparous women with a BS of < 4

        - 2mg gel every 6 hours for 3 doses until BS is 7 or more
    - all multiparous women with a BS of < 4
        - 1mg gel initially and then 2 mg every 6 hours for 3 doses until BS is 7 or more

Syntocinon

- Fluid regime whilst on Syntocinon infusion
    - commence 5% Dextrose in saline solution (if not available use normal saline) at 250ml/hr throughout labour unless contraindicated
- Syntocinon infusion
    - an infusion of 30 IU Syntocinon in 500ml (60 units in 1 litre) of normal saline should be prepared and infused using an infusion pump

Standard regime for all women – Syntocinon infusion

	Time after starting (minutes)	**1milliunit/minute = 1ml/hr**
Initial dose	0	1ml/hr
Increase infusion rate every 30 minutes if contractions are not present or are inadequate.	30	2
	60	4
	90	8
	120	12
	150	16
	180	20

Prior to exceeding 20 milliunits/minute consult with the obstetrician

	Time after starting (minutes)	**1 milliunit/minute = 1ml/hr**
After infusion has been maintained at 20mIU/min for 30 minutes, increase it every 30 minutes until the contractions are adequate.	210	24ml/hr
	240	28
	270	32

Hyperstimulation

Note definitions

Tachysystole: more than 5 contractions in 10 minutes, averaged over a 30-minute window

Hypertonicity: contraction lasting at least 2 minutes

It is hyperstimulation if either of the above occur with FHR abnormality

- Remove the pessary from the vagina if the woman is on a maternity ward
- If in a birth suite
    - stop or reduce the Syntocinon infusion while reassessing labour and the fetal state
    - lie the woman in a left lateral position
    - recommend tocolysis
        - Terbutaline: 250 micrograms subcutaneously

Recommended Reading

1. Du H, Zhang N, Xiao CY et al. Effectiveness of Dinoprostone and Cook's Balloon for Labor Induction in Primipara Women at Term. *Curr. Med. Sci.* 2020 Oct; 40(5): 951-959.
2. Wagner S, Sandoval G, Grobman WA. Labor Induction at 39 Weeks Compared with Expectant Management in Low-Risk Parous Women. *Am. J. Perinatol.* 2020 Sep 11. doi: 10.1055/s-0040-1716711.
3. Bhide A, Sedgwick P, Barrett B et al. Pilot Feasibility Study. 2020 Aug 15; 6: 113.
4. Simpson KR. Cervical Ripening and Labor Induction and Augmentation. *Nurs. Womens. Health.* 2020 Aug; 24(4): S1-S41.
5. Dong S, Khan M, Hashimi F et al. Inpatient versus outpatient induction of labour: a systematic review and meta-analysis. *BMC Pregnancy Childbirth.* 2020 Jun 30; 20(1): 382. doi: 10.1186/s12884-020-03060-1.
6. Levine LD, Valencia CM, Tolosa JE et al. Induction of labor in continuing pregnancies. *Best Pract. Res. Clin. Obstet. Gynaecol.* 2020 Aug; 67: 90-99.
7. Coates D, Makris A, Catling C et al. A systematic scoping review of clinical indications for induction of labour. *PLoS One.* 2020 Jan 29; 15(1): e0228196.

CHAPTER THIRTY-FIVE

INFLAMMATORY BOWEL DISEASE

Ulcerative colitis and Crohn's disease

- Both have periods of relapse and remission
- Ulcerative colitis
  - 30% may flare up in pregnancy
  - it affects only the colon
  - the woman may get abdominal pain with diarrhoea or urgency of defaecation
  - she may pass blood and mucous per rectum
  - complications include
    - toxic megacolon
    - malignancy
    - thromboembolism
- Crohn's disease
  - 15% may flare up
  - affects the terminal ileum, colon, or both, but can affect any part of the gastro intestinal tract from the mouth to the anus
  - abdominal pain is more cramping and often there is weight loss
  - complications include
    - perforation of the bowel
    - strictures and intermittent intestinal obstruction
    - perianal fistulae, abscess
    - malabsorption
    - thromboembolism

Diagnosis – this is often already known

Effect of pregnancy on Inflammatory Bowel Disease (IBD)

- If the disease was quiescent at the time of conception, it will remain so in two thirds of cases
- 30% will get relapses in pregnancy

- Women with active IBD at the time of conception have the highest risk of a relapse
- Ulcerative colitis exacerbation usually occurs in the first two trimesters and are often mild
- Relapses can also occur postpartum

Effect of IBD on pregnancy

- The majority of women will have a full-term normal pregnancy
- There is an increased risk of miscarriage and preterm birth with the active disease
- They may have malabsorption and the risks associated with it
- There may be fetal growth restriction

Management

- Multidisciplinary approach
- Ideally recommend planning conception during a quiescent phase
- If they smoke, advise that they cease (it is associated with worsening disease and more relapses – especially with Crohn's disease)
- Recommend a high dose of folic acid peri conceptually and throughout pregnancy especially if they are on Sulphasalazine
- Advise that she continue to take her IBD medication during the pregnancy – all of them are safe during pregnancy and lactation
- She may need iron and vitamin supplementation
- Recommend Vitamin D supplementation
- Monitor fetal growth and wellbeing
- Treat relapses aggressively
- If on steroids – monitor for glucose intolerance (GDM) and recommend intravenous injection of 100mg Hydrocortisone 6-8 hourly in labour
- There is an increased risk of thromboembolism, particularly if the disease is active
    - recommend thromboprophylaxis
- Aim for a vaginal birth
- Advise on a caesarean section (CS) if she has an active perianal disease, perianal scarring, anal incontinence, or rectovaginal fistulae
    - induction of labour and a caesarean section are otherwise indicated only for obstetric indications

Postpartum

- The risk of flare up is increased in women with active disease in the last few weeks of pregnancy

- Advise her to continue all her IBD medication
- It is safe to breast feed (it may reduce the risk of the baby developing IBD in later life)
- Advise her on appropriate contraception – avoid the combined pill due to its increased risk of thromboembolism in these cases

Recommended Reading

1. Huang V, et al. Management of Inflammatory Bowel Disease in Pregnancy: A Practical Approach to New Guidelines. *Can. J. Gastroenterol. Hepatol*. 2016. PMID: 27478821.
2. Kubota-Sjogren Y. Inflammatory bowel disease in pregnancy: management strategy based on best evidence and European guidelines. *Br. J. Gen. Pract*. 2014. PMID: 25348990.
3. Szymańska E. Reproduction and Pregnancy in Inflammatory Bowel Disease - Management and Treatment Based on Current Guidelines. *J. Gynecol. Obstet. Hum. Reprod*. 2020.
4. Poturoglu S, Ormeci AC, Duman AE. Treatment of pregnant women with a diagnosis of inflammatory bowel disease. *World J. Gastrointest. Pharmacol. Ther*. 2016 Nov 6; 7(4): 490-502.

CHAPTER THIRTY-SIX

LABOUR

Confirm onset of established labour on arrival

- Explain all procedures prior to their being performed
- Keep the woman and her partner informed of the labour progress AND fetal condition at all times
- Involve them in the decision making as much as possible
- Ensure there is a 1:1 woman to midwife ratio
- If a vaginal examination is required:
    - explain the need first
    - Entonox may help if she is anxious or too uncomfortable
- Avoid admitting women to the birthing suite if they're not in true labour. The first stage of labour is the latent phase; it has been defined traditionally as the cervix < 4cm dilated but more recent data suggest cervix < 6cm dilatation
    - check on the baby and advise the woman to go home if all is well with clear instructions as to when to call back or come in
        - she may take Paracetamol 1g 4-6 hourly for pain
    - if she is in too much pain, offer Codeine and observe her in the ward. Repeat a vaginal examination after 4 hours to assess for any change on cervical dilatation

Ambulation in labour

- In the first stage of labour, encourage women to be ambulant
- Encourage the use of showers, and sitting on a chair and rubber ball
- If she desires to be on the bed, encourage her to lie on her side or be well propped up

Fluids and oral intake

- For normal risk women allow food (preferably light food) and fluids in normal labour

- If she is an at-risk woman with a higher than average chance of requiring a CS, recommend drinking clear energy drinks only
- If she has an epidural, advise her to have only clear fluids – restrict opaque fluids and particulate foods

Social support

- A positively motivated support person will promote a satisfying and less interventional birthing process
- Continuity of care is also of benefit

Fetal heart rate monitoring

- In normal risk women one may use intermittent doppler auscultation of the fetal heart rate if labour is progressing normally
    - listen at least every 30 minutes in the first stage, every 5 minutes in the second stage and after every contraction in the second stage if actively pushing
- The following are some of the recommendations for continuous electronic FHR monitoring:
- **antenatal factors:**
    - abnormal doppler umbilical artery velocimetry
    - abnormal antenatal CTG
    - oligohydramnios
    - prolonged pregnancy (> 42 weeks)
    - multiple pregnancy
    - breech presentation
    - antepartum haemorrhage (more than a 'show' or > 50ml)
    - prolonged rupture of membranes (> 24 hours)
    - known fetal abnormality which requires monitoring
    - presence of a uterine scar
    - pre-eclampsia (current pregnancy)
    - gestational diabetes on insulin or poorly controlled diabetes mellitus in pregnancy
    - other medical conditions that constitute a significant risk of fetal compromise

Intra partum factors

- Syntocinon infusion
- epidural analgesia
- vaginal bleeding in labour (more than a 'show' or > 50ml)
- maternal pyrexia
- meconium or blood-stained liquor

  - oligohydramnios or absence of liquor at amniotomy
  - multiple pregnancy
  - active first stage of labour > 12 hours (i.e., regular uterine activity, cervix $\geq$ 4cm dilated)
  - prolonged second stage
  - abnormal FHR on intermittent doppler
- Continuous fetal heart rate monitoring may be performed using an external transducer in women with normal BMI
  - if unable to get a good trace, use a fetal scalp electrode to monitor FH
- Telemetry may allow some women to be mobile and still be monitored continuously

Antibiotics in labour

- These are recommended if
  - she is at risk for EOGBSD or endometritis
  - she has cardiac abnormalities requiring prophylactic antibiotics

Pain relief in labour

- Social support in labour is very helpful
- Consider simple things such as lighting, noise, music etc. if she wishes
- Consider mobilisation and use of showers
- Other modalities include:
  - sterile water injection
  - TENS machine
  - water immersion
  - nitrous oxide (Entonox)
  - opiates – morphine
  - Fentanyl PCA
  - epidural

Monitoring progress in labour – the partogram

- Record all observations on the partogram from the time the woman is admitted in established labour
- If a woman is undergoing induction of labour, commence a partogram at the time of commencement of Syntocinon or at the commencement of labour
- Perform a vaginal examination every 4 hours if progress is normal and every 2 hours if not normal

- The active phase of labour begins at 3-4cm cervical dilatation – though recent data suggest it may be at 6cm dilatation
- Draw an action line once in the active phase of labour
- Generally, expect cervical dilatation to occur at 0.5cm per hour
- It has been shown that primiparous compared to multiparous women may dilate at a slower rate until they reach 6cm
- If progress of labour is slow – attempt to identify the reason and consider:
    - cervical dystocia
    - cephalopelvic disproportion
    - malposition
    - inefficient uterine activity
- Recommend amniotomy if membranes are still intact
- Recommend Syntocinon infusion – especially in primiparous women who may be having strong palpable contractions but which are incoordinate and thus inefficient
- Recommend an epidural analgesia
- When assessing cervical dilatation also assess the level of the presenting part and presence or absence of any caput or moulding
- Assess maternal hydration – use a Hartmann's or saline solution to keep her well hydrated. Some data suggest a 5% dextrose in saline infusion may shorten duration of labour
- Assess fetal wellbeing

Syntocinon in labour

- As noted above it may be required to augment labour which is progressing slowly
    - use it with extreme caution for slow progress in multiparous women
- Consider carefully the need to augment labour in a woman attempting a vaginal birth after a caesarean section (VBAC)

Pushing

- Second stage:
    - allow the passive descent of the presenting part (the cervix is fully dilated but there are no involuntary expulsive contractions)
        - recommend an hour for descent; it may be longer especially if the woman has an epidural and if mother and baby are comfortable

- active – pushing should ideally only be encouraged once the presenting part is low, provided there is no concern over fetal heart rate
    - nulliparous women may push for up to 2 and multiparous women for 1 hour
    - one may allow an hour longer for both if there is no fetal or maternal concern and there is some descent of presenting part before resorting to any intervention
    - if contractions are weak consider use of Syntocinon in primiparous women and with caution in multiparous women
    - ensure the bladder is empty

Delivery

- Use an intrapartum perineal massage and warm compresses to prevent perineal injury
- Apply light pressure on the baby's head to facilitate flexion and control rapid expulsion
- Guard the perineum to avoid perineal tears
- Control delivery of the shoulders as many of the obstetric anal sphincter tears also occur with rapid expulsion of the shoulders
- Perform delayed cord clamping – 60 seconds or longer until pulsation ceases unless baby needs urgent attention
- Encourage early skin to skin contact
- Encourage early breast feeding

Third stage of labour:

Active management is the standard recommendation

- Some women will choose physiological management
- If a woman is at high risk of postpartum haemorrhage also commence 30 units/500ml saline of Syntocinon infusion at 10 IU/hour
- Examine the placenta and membranes to ensure all are complete
- Examine for perineal trauma
- If she is Rhesus negative consider the need for and dose of anti D immunoglobulin

Recommended Reading

1. Lavender T. Use of the partograph - Current thinking. *Best Pract. Res. Clin. Obstet. Gynaecol.* 2020 Aug; 67:33-43.

2. Nanji JA, Carvalho B.Nanji JA, et al. Pain management during labor and vaginal birth. *Best Pract. Res. Clin. Obstet. Gynaecol.* 2020 Aug; 67: 100-112.
3. Abalos E, Chamillard M, Díaz V et al. Progression of the first stage of spontaneous labour. *Best Pract. Res. Clin. Obstet. Gynaecol.* 2020 Aug; 67: 19-32.
4. Rhoades JS, Cahill AG. Rhoades JS, et al. Defining and Managing Normal and Abnormal First Stage of Labor. *Obstet. Gynecol. Clin. North Am.* 2017 Dec;44(4):535-545.
5. Zhang J, Troendle J, Grantz KL et al. Statistical aspects of modeling the labor curve. *Am. J. Obstet. Gynecol.* 2015 Jun; 212(6): 750.e1-4. doi: 10.1016/j.ajog.2015.04.01.

CHAPTER THIRTY-SEVEN

LISTERIA INFECTION IN PREGNANCY

A food borne infection that is more common in summer – the bacterium Listeria monocytogenes can survive in temperature of 4-degrees Celsius.

- Advise pregnant women to avoid foods such as hot dogs, cold meats served chilled, refrigerated pâté and meat spreads, refrigerated smoked seafood, raw (unpasteurized) milk and unpasteurized soft cheeses
- Advise them to cook food thoroughly and wash salads, fruit, and raw vegetables thoroughly

Clinical features

There may be mild flu like symptoms, backache, vomiting or diarrhoea, muscle pains and sore throat

- About 30% of cases are asymptomatic
- Suspect infection in any pregnant woman with a fever and gastrointestinal symptoms

Effect on pregnancy

- Transmission to the fetus is highest in the third trimester
- Fetal risks include
    - miscarriage or fetal loss (for infections in first trimester)
    - preterm birth
    - intrauterine fetal death – infection in the second and third trimesters carries a fetal mortality rate of 40-50%
    - neonatal Listeriosis:
        - early onset (first 24-48 hours) may result in:
            - septicaemia (81-88%)
            - respiratory distress or pneumonia (38%)
            - meningitis (24%) – typically this occurs in preterm infants
        - late onset (5 days to few weeks postpartum), typically this occurs in term neonates and may result in:
            - placental, cord or pharyngeal granulomas

- papular or pustular skin rash
- conjunctivitis
- septicaemia (17-95%)
- meningitis (67-93%)

Diagnosis

- Diagnosis is made by culture of the gram-positive bacilli from a sterile site such as blood, amniotic fluid or cerebrospinal fluid
    - recommend doing a blood culture in any pregnant woman who presents with fever and flu or gastroenteritis like symptoms
    - vaginal or stool cultures are not helpful in the diagnosis because some women are carriers and do not have the clinical disease
    - placental and other autopsy specimen cultures may also be used to confirm the diagnosis

Management

- If an exposed pregnant woman presents with a fever > 38° and has signs and symptoms consistent with Listeriosis and no other cause to explain the illness
    - recommend doing a blood culture
    - treat simultaneously for Listeriosis - Amoxicillin/Ampicillin 2g 4-6 hourly and Gentamicin 80mg daily intravenously for 14 days
    - recommend urgent delivery depending on gestation and maternal condition
- In asymptomatic women at high risk of Listeriosis who have ingested food implicated in an outbreak, consider treating them with oral Amoxicillin, 2-3g daily for 7 days
- Recommend screening neonates:
    - send placenta for culture
    - request superficial swabs, blood culture, urine and CSF for culture and gram stain
    - chest X ray to exclude pneumonia
        - recommend empiric treatment with Amoxycillin/Ampicillin (50mg/kg) and Gentamicin (2.5mg/kg) twice daily for 2-3 weeks
        - if neonate remains well and culture return is negative
            - can cease antibiotics

Recommended Reading

1. Institute of Obstetricians and Gynaecologists, Royal College of Physicians of Ireland and the Clinical Strategy and Programmes Division, Health Service Executive. *Clinical Practice Guideline.* Listeriosis in Pregnancy. Nov 2015.
2. Pucci L, Massacesi M, Liuzzi G. Clinical management of women with listeriosis risk during pregnancy: a review of national guidelines. *Expert Rev. Anti Infect. Ther.* 2018 Jan; 16(1): 13-21.
3. Craig AM, Dotters-Katz S, Kuller JA, Thompson JL Listeriosis in Pregnancy: A Review. *Obstet. Gynecol. Surv.* 2019 Jun; 74(6): 362-368.
4. Rac H, Gould AP, Eiland LS et al. Common Bacterial and Viral Infections: Review of Management in the Pregnant Patient. *Ann Pharmacother.* 2019 Jun; 53(6): 639-651.
5. Palasanthiran P, Starr M, Jones C. Ed: Management of Perinatal Infections. Sydney: Australasian Society for Infectious Diseases (ASID); 2014.

CHAPTER THIRTY-EIGHT

MACROSOMIA

Definition

- Large for gestational age (LGA) is when the estimated fetal weight is > 90th centile. Macrosomia is when the estimated fetal weight (EFW) is > 4.5kg (some say > 4kg)

Incidence

- 10% and it appears to be rising

Risks factors for LGA

- Maternal diabetes and gestational diabetes (GDM)
    - strict control can reduce this risk
- High BMI
- Previous LGA
- Excess weight gain in pregnancy
- Post term > 42 weeks
- Male infant

Risks associated with LGA

- Caesarean section for FTP
- Postpartum haemorrhage
- Shoulder dystocia
- 3rd and 4th degree tears
- Birth trauma – brachial plexus injuries – transient or permanent
- Fractures
- HIE
- Intrauterine and neonatal death

Prevention

- In women with diabetes dietary intervention with addition of insulin reduces likelihood of birthweight > 90th centile

- Control of maternal hyperglycaemia reduces the risk of macrosomia
  - recommend strict maternal glucose control in women with diabetes

Estimating fetal weight

- The ultrasound scan estimation of fetal weight is unreliable
  - it can vary by up to 20%
  - > 30% of fetuses that are LGA on a scan are not so at birth

Management

- There is no consistent approach
  - clinicians generally still use ultrasound scans to rule out macrosomia
- Randomised clinical trials have not shown the clinical effectiveness of prophylactic caesarean section when EFW < 5000g in non-diabetics
- Induction of labour for suspected macrosomia reduces the risk of shoulder dystocia and any type of fracture
  - there is no change in the risk of caesarean section or instrumental delivery
  - there is no difference between the groups with or without induction of labour for brachial plexus injury
- Recommend elective caesarean section
  - if EFW > 4.5kg in a diabetic and > 5kg in a non-diabetic woman
    - 50% of shoulder dystocia (SD) cases occur in babies weighing < 4kg
  - if she had shoulder dystocia in a previous pregnancy with permanent nerve injury
- Also advise women that 30% of nerve injuries occur without shoulder dystocia
  - a significant number of injuries occur antenatally
- Expectant management and awaiting spontaneous onset of labour are also options
  - there is some consensus to offer induction of labour at 38^0-38^6 weeks if
    - EFW is > 3500g at 36 weeks
    - EFW is > 3700g at 37 weeks
    - EFW is > 3900g at 38 weeks
- In all women with slow progress of labour, maintain a heightened awareness for SD

Recommended Reading

1. J Beta 1, N Khan 1, M Fiolna et al. Maternal and neonatal complications of fetal macrosomia: cohort study *Ultrasound Obstet. Gynecol.* 2019 Sep; 54(3): 319-325.
2. Akanmode AM, Mahdy H. Macrosomia. 2020 Aug 23. In: StatPearls [Internet]. Treasure Island (FL): StatPearls Publishing; 2020 Jan– PMID: 32491509.
3. Macrosomia ACOG Practice Bulletin, Number 216, *Obstetrics & Gynecology*: January 2020 - Volume 135 - Issue 1 - p e18-e35.
4. Robinson R, Walker KF, White VA et al. The test accuracy of antenatal ultrasound definitions of fetal macrosomia to predict birth injury: A systematic review. *Eur. J. Obstet. Gynecol. Reprod. Biol.* 2020 Mar; 246: 79-85.

CHAPTER THIRTY-NINE

MECONIUM STAINING OF THE LIQUOR

Meconium staining of the liquor (MSL) occurs in 10% of all pregnancies and may reflect gastrointestinal tract (GIT) maturity.

- Meconium may be passed from 10 weeks gestation, but it is uncommon to see MSL before 34 weeks
- Incidence of MSL in labour increases with increasing gestational age (30% at 40 weeks and 50% at 42 weeks)
- **Meconium aspiration (MAS)**
    - the risk increases with increasing gestational age
    - clinical disease ranges from mild transient respiratory distress to severe respiratory compromise requiring prolonged mechanical ventilation
    - it is not independently associated with any long-term neurological abnormality
    - it used to be thought that meconium aspiration occurred at time of birth with the first breath but now it's thought to be a predominantly intrauterine event
    - meconium aspiration is more common with thick meconium than with thin meconium – probably because it is associated with oligohydramnios (thick undiluted meconium)

Management in labour

- Recommend continuous electronic fetal heart rate (FHR) monitoring
- Amnio-infusion may have some benefit in reducing variable decelerations and in turn risk of caesarean section in women with thick meconium
    - possibly by diluting the meconium and/or reducing oligohydramnios
    - probably only of value in under resourced countries where FBS facility may not be available
- Avoid incidences which may provoke hypoxia
    - avoid supine hypotension
    - avoid uterine hyper-stimulation with Syntocinon

- There is no need for routine fetal blood sampling in labour if FHR is normal

Delivery

- Request Paediatrician to be present at birth
    - if the baby is vigorous and cries, there is no need for any action
    - if the baby is born with respiratory depression, heart rate < 100bpm, or is floppy – **do not vigorously stimulate the baby**.
        - recommend endometrial suctioning under direct vision
        - the degree of meconium thickness independently correlates with the composite adverse neonatal outcome

Recommended Reading

1. Sayad E, Silva-Carmona M. Meconium Aspiration. 2020 May 24. In: StatPearls [Internet]. Treasure Island (FL): StatPearls Publishing; 2020 Jan–.PMID: 32491357.
2. Kelly T. Fetal distress in labor. In: *Evidence Based Obstetrics*, Ed. James DK, 5th edition. WB Saunders UK. 2017.
3. Phattraprayoon N, Tangamornsuksan W, Ungtrakul T. Outcomes of endotracheal suctioning in non-vigorous neonates born through meconium-stained amniotic fluid: a systematic review and meta-analysis. *Arch. Dis. Child Fetal Neonatal Ed.* 2021 Jan; 106(1): 31-38.
4. Gluck O, Kovo M, Tairy D et al. The effect of meconium thickness level on neonatal outcome. *Early Hum. Dev.* 2020 Mar; 142: 104953.

CHAPTER FORTY

MISCARRIAGE

Miscarriage occurs in 20% of pregnancies.

Risk factors for miscarriage include

- Chromosomal abnormalities that are found in 60% of cases
    - Trisomy, Monosomy X and Triploidy are the commonest chromosomal abnormalities
- Demographic risk factors
    - advanced maternal age, high BMI, black ethnicity
- Lifestyle risk factors
    - smoking, alcohol and substance use, high caffeine intake
- Clinical risk factors
    - antiphospholipid antibodies, thyroid disorders, congenital uterine anomalies and uterine septae
- Infections
    - Bacterial Vaginosis, Brucellosis, Chlamydia Trachomatis, Syphilis, Herpes viruses infection, Cytomegalovirus, Human Papilloma virus, Parvovirus, Hepatitis B and C and Toxoplasmosis infections

Threatened miscarriage

- Vaginal bleeding is often slight (usually less than a normal period) and painless
- On examination the internal os of the cervix is closed
- Depending on the gestational age fetal cardiac activity may be detectable on a scan

Inevitable miscarriage

- Bleeding is heavier and associated with cramping pain over the uterus
- The internal os is open
- Products of conception may be visible in the cervix

Incomplete miscarriage

- Bleeding may be heavy with clots and she may have noticed products of conception
- There is often cramping and lower abdominal pain
- The internal os of the cervix is open and products of conception may be visible in the cervix
- This may be complicated by hypovolaemic shock and or sepsis with pyrexia and lower abdominal tenderness

Complete miscarriage

- The entire contents of the uterus may be expelled resulting in a complete miscarriage

Missed miscarriage

- The fetus has died but products have not yet been expelled
- The woman may complain of brown vaginal discharge
- Symptoms of pregnancy may have disappeared
- On examination the internal os is closed

Examination should include assessment of

- General condition
  - vital signs (tachycardia usually precedes hypotension in acute haemorrhage in young women)
  - look for any evidence of infection
  - there may be postural hypotension
- Perform a speculum examination
  - to see the source of bleeding
  - to exclude obvious products of conception in the cervical os
    - if visible, use a sponge holder to gently remove them
- The presence of cervical motion tenderness may suggest sepsis or an ectopic pregnancy

Useful ultrasound findings

- In early pregnancy failure there may be a gestational sac with diameter of > 20mm with no yolk sac or a gestational sac of > 25mm with no fetal pole
- In a missed miscarriage/fetal demise there may be a fetal pole of ≥ 6mm with no cardiac activity
  - cardiac activity should always be present in a normally developing embryo with a crown rump length (CRL) of 6mm or more

  - if the CRL is 7mm or more with a transvaginal scan and there is no cardiac activity, repeat the scan a minimum of 7 days after the first before making a diagnosis of missed miscarriage
  - if there is a gestational sac on a transvaginal scan but no visible fetal pole, it is safer to repeat the scan a minimum of 7 days later before making a diagnosis of missed miscarriage
- If bleeding is not marked and there is uncertainty about retained products of conception, an ultrasound scan will often show heterogenous shadow within the endometrial cavity; if this is less than 15mm, it is unlikely that surgical evacuation is necessary and should be avoided

Management of a woman with bleeding in early pregnancy
- Resuscitate if required
- Check Rhesus group:
  - if she's Rh negative – recommend anti D immunoglobulin
- Consider a blood culture if she's febrile
- Recommend analgesia as needed – non-steroidal anti-inflammatory drugs (NSAIDs) are best avoided

Threatened miscarriage – manage expectantly with reassurance. There is no evidence to support restricting physical activity except advising to avoid vaginal intercourse
- There is no benefit from hospital admission
- If bleeding settles, an ultrasound scan may be repeated in about 7 days

All other miscarriages with heavy vaginal bleeding
- If products of conception are protruding from the cervical os, remove them and see if this reduces bleeding
- Administer Ergometrine (500mcg intramuscularly)
- You can also give an intramuscular injection of 5-10 units of Syntocinon or 1000mcg of Misoprostol via the rectum to reduce blood loss
- Most women will need to go to theatre for suction curettage if the bleeding is heavy

All other miscarriages where vaginal bleeding is not very heavy
- Discuss expectant, medical, and surgical management – all of these options have been shown to be safe

Surgical management

- Use a soft Carmen cannula for the suction as its use is associated with less blood loss and a lower risk of perforation
- Perform a vaginal examination to assess the size of the uterus but more importantly to make sure it is not retroverted
    - if it is retroverted apply valsellum forceps to the anterior lip of the cervix and apply downward traction to antevert it while introducing the cannula
- Use a cannula size that is 2mm smaller than the size of the uterus in weeks
- Very gently insert the cannula, holding it between thumb and index finger into the uterine cavity
- Attach it then to the suction tubing
- Keep in mind the markers that show the position of the curetting edge and use the index finger to apply pressure against the uterine wall when suctioning
- Perform suction by gentle rotation as well as an in and out action (rotation is generally required to dislodge tissue in women with a missed miscarriage)
- Do this methodically at 12, 3, 6 and 9 o'clock and avoid taking the cannula in and out of the uterus too often except if you suspect that the cannula may be blocked with tissue
- Stop as soon as complete evacuation has occurred
- Complete evacuation has occurred if:
    - the cervix clamps over the cannula
    - you only see air bubbles in the cannula and tubing
    - you feel a gritty sensation
- There is no need to then use a sharp curette as this only increases the risk of perforation
- If bleeding is heavy, recommend Syntometrine or Ergometrine as first line drugs
- Send all tissue for histology to exclude ectopic pregnancy and gestational trophoblastic disease
- In cases where suction curettage is required with a closed cervix, recommend using 400ug Misoprostol vaginally or orally 3-4 hours prior to surgery
- In all at risk women undergoing surgical evacuation, screen for Chlamydia Trachomatis, especially in women under the age of 25 years
- Prophylactic antibiotics are not normally indicated

- Advise her to maintain pelvic rest (nothing should be inserted in the vagina) for 2 weeks, at which time coitus and the use of tampons may be resumed
- It has been traditional to advise that pregnancy be deferred for 2-3 months although there does not appear to be any evidence of adverse outcome with shorter intervals

Medical management up to 18 weeks – option 1

- Bleeding will last longer than surgical management and the surgical option may be necessary if bleeding gets heavier or is persistent beyond a reasonable time
- Recommend anti-Progesterone (Mifepristone) 200mcg on day 1
- On day 2 or 3 recommend 400mcg oral or vaginal Misoprostol
- On day 4, repeat the dose of 400mcg unless a complete miscarriage is confirmed
- On day 8, review and repeat hCG levels to ensure the level is dropping
    - consider suction curettage if there is ongoing heavy bleeding
- Do a final review 6 weeks after the first dose of Misoprostol

Medical management up to 18 weeks – option 2

- Recommend Misoprostol 400mcg every 3 or every 6 hours (vaginal or sublingual)
- She may require more than 3 doses

Expectant management

- As long as her vital signs are stable and there is no evidence of infection, this "wait and see" approach may be considered if bleeding is not excessive
- All cases of expectant management should be followed up weekly in the early pregnancy clinic until symptoms have resolved and hCG levels drop to less than 2IU/L
- During expectant management the woman may get heavy bleeding when tissue is passed. She must have easy access to a telephone and to emergency services if bleeding becomes heavy in which case she may need to go to theatre for suction curettage
    - 40 % of women on expectant management end up having a suction curettage
- Arrange a follow-up scan at 7-10 days
    - if there still is bleeding, pain or evidence of retained products of conception, discuss options for continued expectant, medical or surgical management

Anti-D immunoprophylaxis

- Recommend anti-D immunoglobulin (250IU) for all non-sensitised Rh-negative women who present with any form of miscarriage
- Cytogenetic assessment of tissue is usually only requested with ≥ 3 recurrent miscarriages

Psychological aspects of early pregnancy loss

- Miscarriage may be associated with significant psychological sequelae. Recommend social worker support
- Offer an opportunity to attend a follow up clinic in 2 weeks

Recommended Reading

1. Clinical Practice Guidelines for Early Pregnancy Loss – Qld Maternal, Neonatal and Gynaecology Clinical Service Network. May 2017.
2. Miscarriage - Management - Approach - Best Practice – BMJ Best Practice; 2016.
3. Petersen SG, Perkins AR, Gibbons KS et al. The medical management of missed miscarriage: outcomes from a prospective, single-centre, Australian cohort. *Med. J. Aust.* 2013; 199 (5): 341-346.
4. Quenby S, Gallos ID, Dhillon-Smith RK et al. Miscarriage matters: the epidemiological, physical, psychological, and economic costs of early pregnancy loss. *Lancet*. 2021 May 1; 397(10285): 1658-1667.

CHAPTER FORTY-ONE

MULTIPLE PREGNANCY

Twin births account for about 3% of live births.

- Dizygotic or "fraternal" twins occur from ovulation and fertilization of two oocytes
  - most of these are DCDA twins
- Monozygotic or "identical" twins result from ovulation and fertilization of a single oocyte, with subsequent division of the zygote
  - division in < 3 days may result in DCDA (30%)
  - division during 4–7 days may result in monochorionic, diamniotic (MCDA) (70%)
  - division during 8–12 days may result in monochorionic, monoamniotic (MCMA) (< 1%)
  - division occurring > 12 days later may result in conjoined twins (very rare)

Early scan

- Allows for early identification, accurate dating and documenting type of twin pregnancy
- Also helps to exclude severe fetal malformation

Risks due to multiple pregnancy

Fetal

- Preterm delivery < 32 weeks (1% singleton versus 5% with twins)
- Fetal growth restriction (MCDA > DCDA)
- Congenital malformations (with monochorionic twins)
- Higher rate of stillbirth
- Increased perinatal mortality and long-term neonatal morbidity especially with MCDA twins

Maternal

- Exaggerated symptoms of pregnancy
- Increased risk of miscarriage (more with MCDA than DCDA)
- Anaemia

- Hypertension – gestational hypertension and preeclampsia (similar risk with MCDA and DCDA)
- Placental abruption
- Gestational diabetes
- Acute fatty liver
- Thromboembolism
- Obstetric cholestasis
- PUPP
- Postpartum haemorrhage
- Higher maternal mortality

MC twins in addition are at increased risk of

- Twin-twin transfusion syndrome (TTTS) – seen in 10-15% of monochorionic twin pregnancies
    - there is oligohydramnios (DVP < 2cm) in one amniotic sac and polyhydramnios (DVP > 8cm if under 20 weeks and > 10cm if over 20 weeks) in the other sac
    - it can also occur in monochorionic and dichorionic triplets and thus terminology is feto-fetal transfusion syndrome (FFTS)
    - 20% of stillbirths are due to FFTS
- Twin anaemia-polycythaemia sequence (TAPS) – one twin is anaemic and the other twin is polycythaemic, but without amniotic fluid volume discordance
- Twin reversed arterial perfusion sequence (TRAP) – the live twin perfuses a non-alive twin
- Selective fetal growth restriction – the weight of one twin is below the 10th percentile or there is discordance in growth; weight difference is greater than 25% (weight of larger twin – weight of smaller twin) ÷ weight of larger twin, expressed as a percentage
- Single fetal demise
    - in DCDA
        - there is then an increased risk of preterm birth with the ongoing pregnancy with the second twin
        - there is a 5-10% risk of stillbirth and cerebral palsy in the surviving twin
    - in MCDA
        - there is a 30% risk of stillbirth and neurological handicap

Monoamniotic twins – there is a risk of cord entanglement and conjoined twins

Management
Preferably by a dedicated team
Antenatal

- Ensure continuity of care
- Ensure a multidisciplinary approach for social and emotional support
- Recommend peri conceptual folic acid and a well-balanced diet
- Recommend iron and folic acid supplementation till birth
    - monitor Hb levels to detect anaemia early
- Recommend Aspirin 150mg at bedtime and calcium 600mg twice daily to prevent PIH from 7 weeks (this can start at any time up to 16 weeks gestation and continue till 36 weeks)
- Assess for VTE risk at each visit
- Recommend first trimester screen
    - confirm gestational age
        - use the CRL of the largest of the fetuses to calculate gestational age
    - exclude major congenital malformation
    - determine chorionicity
        - in dichorionic twins
            - there may be two separate placentae
            - the inter-twin membrane is thicker (absent in monochorionic twins)
            - there may be a twin peak sign (or a "T' sign or lambda sign) – this is a triangular projection of tissue that extends between layers of the intertwin membrane from a fused dichorionic placenta; it is best seen at 10 to 14 weeks
                - after 20 weeks only 85% of DCDA twins will show a lambda sign
            - different sexes seen later in pregnancy
        - in monochorionic twins
            - absence of "T" sign on intertwin membrane – appearance of the thin intertwin membrane composed of two amnions as it takes off from the placenta at a 90-degree angle
- Non-invasive prenatal testing (NIPT)
    - this is a poor test in multiple pregnancy as there is less cell free DNA and the cell free DNA is derived from each of the 2 twins
    - there is also a high false positive rate

- Recommend a morphology scan at around 20 weeks (request cervical length as well)
- Repeat the scan to assess cervical length at 24 weeks – it may be used to guide use of progesterone to reduce the risk of preterm birth
    - **see chapter on preterm birth for possible interventions to prevent preterm birth**
- Monitor growth
    - dichorionic twins – scan every 4 weeks and more frequently if there is discordant growth
    - monochorionic twins – scan at 16 weeks and then every 2 weeks until birth
        - offer an initial scan preferably at a tertiary centre or by an MFM specialist
        - all scans should be at a tertiary centre if there is any evidence of FFTS
            - plot all scan measurements on a growth chart and see the trend in growth
        - assess growth discordance:
            - monitor as for FGR
            - recommend a weekly AFI and doppler if
                - growth discordance is 20% or more
                - the EFW of any of the babies is < 10th centile
- Monitor for onset of pre-eclampsia
    - check blood pressure and urine at each visit
- Assess fetal wellbeing (only if FGR is confirmed)
- **At the 32-34 weeks visit**
    - discuss timing and mode of birth
        - there is a 60% risk of spontaneous preterm labour in twins
        - there is a 70% risk of preterm birth < 35 weeks in triplets
    - discuss care in labour
- In threatened preterm labour fetal fibronectin testing is as reliable a negative predictor as it is in singleton pregnancies

Triplets

- There is a greater likelihood of Down's syndrome, Edwards' syndrome and Patau's syndrome in triplet pregnancy

- There is increased false positive rate of screening tests in triplet pregnancy
- The woman has a greater likelihood of being offered invasive testing and of complications as a result of it
- There are physical risks and psychological implications in the short and long term when relating fetal reduction is performed
    - o assess growth discordance
        - (EFW largest fetus − EFW smallest fetus) ÷ EFW largest fetus and
        - (EFW largest fetus − EFW middle fetus) ÷ EFW largest fetus, all expressed as a percentage .

Timing of delivery

- DCDA twins – perinatal mortality is increased after 38 weeks; if there is normal growth, recommend delivery at 38^0-38^6 weeks and earlier if there is any concern
- MCDA twins – various guidelines recommend different gestational ages for delivery (generally recommend delivering at 37^0-37^6 weeks if growth is absolutely normal)
    - o deliver at 36^0 if there are any concerns
- TCTA – deliver at 35^6 with steroid loading 7 days prior
- MCMA – deliver at 33^6 with steroid loading 7 days prior
    - o if she declines early delivery, see weekly for AFI, umbilical artery doppler and CTG

Mode of delivery

- If the leading twin is vertex, it is safe for mother and baby to aim for a vaginal delivery
    - o sub analysis of data from twin birth study suggests this may be so for gestational age < 37 weeks and that for twins at ≥ 37 weeks the outcome may be better with a caesarean section
- If the leading twin is non vertex – discuss options of caesarean section or vaginal breech delivery

Labour

- Notify the paediatrician, anaesthetist and theatre
- Insert a cannula for access and send blood for group and hold
- Recommend epidural analgesia once in labour to assist with the delivery of the second twin or if an emergency caesarean section is required
- Recommend continuous fetal heart rate monitoring of both twins during labour

    - apply a fetal scalp electrode onto the leading cephalic twin if 34 weeks
    - if FHR is concerning
        - lactate if 34 weeks
- Ensure the consultant is present at delivery

After delivery of the first twin

Assess presentation of the second twin

- If the presentation is breech or transverse, attempt an ECV or internal podalic version
- If the fetus is cephalic or turns to cephalic after the ECV
    - continue FHR monitoring
    - rupture membranes if they're intact during a contraction
    - if contractions are poor, commence a Syntocinon infusion
    - wait for spontaneous vaginal birth as long as there is no concern about FHR
        - if there is any concern about FHR expedite the birth by which ever mode that is indicated
- If the fetus remains breech or transverse
    - perform an assisted breech delivery if there is the spontaneous rupture of membranes and the breech is low in the pelvis
    - perform a breech extraction for most and aim to deliver within 30 minutes
        - locate the fetal foot/feet
        - grasp one or both feet and apply gentle traction
        - perform an amniotomy whilst traction is being applied

Third stage

- Recommend active management
- Recommend a Syntocinon infusion for 4 hours to maintain uterine contraction
- Send the placenta fresh to confirm chorionicity

Postnatal

- Offer a longer inpatient stay if needed
- Arrange support at home
- Link with multiple pregnancy support groups
- Discuss contraception

Recommended Reading

1. Gibson JL, Castleman JS, Meher S, Kilby MD. Updated guidance for the management of twin and triplet pregnancies from the National Institute for Health and Care Excellence guidance, UK: What's new that may improve perinatal outcomes? *Acta. Obstet. Gynecol. Scand.* 2020 Feb; 99(2): 147-152.
2. Tsakiridis I, Giouleka S, Mamopoulos A et al. Management of Twin Pregnancies: A Comparative Review of National and International Guidelines. *Obstet. Gynecol. Surv.* 2020 Jul; 75(7): 419-430.
3. Axelsdóttir Í, Ajne G. Short-term outcome of the second twin during vaginal delivery is dependent on delivery time interval but not chorionicity. *J. Obstet. Gynaecol.* 2019 Apr; 39(3): 308-312.
4. Zafman KB, Naqvi M, Melka S et al. The Association between Intended Mode of Delivery and Maternal Morbidity in Twin Pregnancies. *Am. J. Perinatol.* 2019 Jun; 36(7): 695-700.
5. Khalil A, Beune I, Hecher K et al. Consensus definition and essential reporting parameters of selective fetal growth restriction in twin pregnancy: a Delphi procedure. *Ultrasound Obstet. Gynecol.* 2019 Jan; 53(1): 47-54.
6. Lipworth H, Hiersch L, Farine D et al. Current Practice of Maternal-Fetal Medicine Specialists Regarding the Prevention and Management of Preterm Birth in Twin Gestations. *J. Obstet. Gynaecol. Can.* 2020 Nov 20: S1701-2163.
7. Behrendt N, Galan HL. Fetal Growth in Multiple Gestations: Evaluation and Management. *Obstet. Gynecol. Clin. North Am.* 2021 Jun; 48(2): 401-417.
8. Couck I, Ponnet S, Thewissen L et al. The Detection, Outcome, and Presentation of Twin-Twin Transfusion Syndrome in Monochorionic Diamniotic Twin Pregnancies Followed with a Protocol of Fortnightly Ultrasound Examination. *Fetal Diagn. Ther.* 2021; 48(5): 353-360.
9. Ochsenbein-Kölble N. Twin pregnancies. *Ultraschall Med.* 2021 Jun; 42(3): 246-269.
10. Ding G, Vinturache A, Yu J et al. Optimal delivery timing for twin pregnancies: A population-based retrospective cohort study. *Int. J. Clin. Pract.* 2021 May; 75(5): e14014.
11. Zork N, Gulersen M, Mardy A et al. The utility of fetal fibronectin in asymptomatic singleton and twin pregnancies with a cervical length 10 mm. *J. Matern. Fetal Neonatal Med.* 2020 Sep; 33(17): 2865-2871.

CHAPTER FORTY-TWO

NAUSEA AND VOMITING – HYPEREMESIS GRAVIDARUM

50-70% of women will have some degree of nausea and vomiting in pregnancy, usually from about 6 weeks and ending by 20 weeks in 90% of cases.

Hyperemesis gravidarum (HG) is the severe form of nausea and vomiting of pregnancy.

- It affects about 0.05 to 1% of pregnancies
- It usually starts at around 6-8 weeks gestation
- Asian women have higher rates
- Features include:
    - excessive vomiting
    - weight loss exceeding 5% of pre-pregnancy body weight
    - evidence of dehydration and electrolyte imbalance
    - ketonuria unrelated to other causes
    - postural hypotension
    - tachycardia

Other conditions that cause nausea and vomiting in pregnancy

- Urinary tract infection
- Gastroenteritis
- Cholecystitis
- Drug induced vomiting
- Hepatitis
- Pancreatitis
- Addison's disease

Obtain detailed history including any maternal disease or conditions related to nausea and vomiting

- Nausea and vomiting in previous pregnancy
- Quantify severity
- Exclude other causes
- Examine for dehydration, muscle wasting, and weight loss

Investigations

- Ward urinalysis for ketones
- Mid-stream urine (MSU) for culture
- Monitor electrolytes – hypokalaemia, hyponatraemia and hypochloraemic metabolic alkalosis
- full blood count – raised haematocrit from haemoconcentration
- abnormal thyroid function test – biochemical hyperthyroidism
    - does not require treatment
    - resolves spontaneously as hyperemesis improves
- Liver enzymes are moderately elevated in 50% of cases who are admitted to hospital – ALT is elevated more than AST; there may be elevated serum bilirubin levels (rarely > 4mg/ml) and mildly elevated amylase levels – all these resolve as HG resolves
- Recommend testing blood sugar level to exclude diabetic ketoacidosis and serum amylase to exclude pancreatitis
- Recommend an ultrasound scan to confirm ongoing pregnancy and exclude multiple pregnancy or hydatidiform mole

Effect on pregnancy

- If left untreated she may develop micronutrient deficiency
- Wernicke encephalopathy (from deficiency of vitamin B1 - thiamine)
    - may be precipitated by excess intravenous Dextrose solution
    - causes blurred vision, drowsiness, and confusion
    - there may be nystagmus, 6th nerve palsy, cerebellar ataxia and hyporeflexia
    - LFTs may be abnormal
        - treat with thiamine (she may not have a complete recovery)
- Hyponatraemia (< 120mmol/l)
    - may cause lethargy, seizures and respiratory arrest
- Oesophageal tears (Mallory-Weiss), oesophageal rupture, pneumothorax and acute tubular necrosis can rarely occur
- Increased risk for thromboembolism

Prevention

- Peri conceptual multivitamin with folic acid decreases the frequency and severity of nausea and vomiting during pregnancy
- Avoidance of triggers
    - stuffy rooms, odours, heat, humidity, noise and visual or physical motion
- Brushing teeth after eating
- Getting enough rest
- Avoid taking iron supplementation in early pregnancy
- Recommend a high carbohydrate, low fat diet in small frequent meals
- Acupuncture
- Ginger powder or ginger containing foods for mild nausea and vomiting

Management

- The earlier the treatment of nausea and vomiting the lesser the chance of developing hyperemesis
- Combination drugs are better than single drug regimens
- Medications that can be used include:
    - Pyridoxine (Vitamin B6): although commonly used it has been shown to be ineffective – 25mg orally every 8 hours
    - Thiamine hydrochloride tabs 25-50mg three times daily
    - Metoclopramide (Maxolon) – 5 to 10mg intravenously or orally (ideally 30 minutes prior to meals and at bedtime) every six hours. Its use is associated with the risk of extra pyramidal signs and oculogyric crises. Keep the max dose to 30mg in 24 hours and avoid its use for more than 5-7 days
    - Promethazine (Avomine): 12.5-25mg – it may cause sedation; it can be given orally, per rectum, intramuscularly, or intravenously (every four hours)
    - Serotonin antagonists — Ondansetron (Selective 5HT3 receptor agonist): 4-8 mg can be taken orally every eight hours, as needed. It can also be administered intravenously every eight hours. It is available as wafers to dissolve in the mouth
        - can cause headache, fatigue, constipation, and drowsiness
    - Phenothiazines (Chlorpromazine and Domperidone)
    - Doxylamine (Restavit) – 25mg tablets, one at night
    - Glucocorticoids – Prednisolone (10mg) orally every eight hours for 2-3 days for refractory cases

Hospitalisation

- Recommend nil orally – introduce clear fluids gradually only after vomiting has stopped after about 24 hours
- A major cause of relapse is the premature introduction of food and fluids
- Intravenous fluids and electrolyte replacement:
    - this is the most important component of management
    - normal saline or Hartmann's solution (avoid glucose as it may precipitate Wernicke's encephalopathy)
    - replace electrolytes as needed
        - monitor for hypokalaemia and hyponatraemia
    - Thiamine supplementation (100mg in 100ml saline over 30 minutes intravenously daily for two or three days) if vomiting for > 3 weeks
- Thromboprophylaxis (Clexane) – can be discontinued upon discharge
- Parenteral nutrition is recommended if she cannot maintain weight because of vomiting and despite a trial of the interventions described above. It is best done via gastric or duodenal intubation rather than the parenteral route
- Give antiemetics as above

Recurrence in subsequent pregnancies

- This can be as high as 50%

Recommended Reading

1. Mullin PM, Ching CY, Schoenberg F et al. Risk factors, treatments, and outcomes associated with prolonged hyperemesis gravidarum. *J. Mater. Fetal Neonatal Med.* 2012; 25(6): 632–636.
2. London V, Grube S, Sherer DM et al. Hyperemesis Gravidarum: A Review of Recent Literature. *Pharmacology*. 2017; 100(3-4): 161-171.
3. Matthews A, Dowswell T, Haas DM et al. Interventions for nausea and vomiting in early pregnancy. *Cochrane Database Syst. Rev.* 2016; (9): CD007575.
4. RCOG. The management of nausea and vomiting of pregnancy and hyperemesis gravidarum. Green-top Guideline No. 69. June 2016.

CHAPTER FORTY-THREE

OBESITY IN PREGNANCY

WHO definition

- Normal weight – BMI ≥ 18.5 to 24.9kg/m^2
- Overweight – BMI ≥ 25 to 29.9kg/m^2
- Obesity class I – BMI 30 to 34.9kg/m^2
- Obesity class II – BMI 35 to 39.9kg/m^2
- Obesity class III – BMI ≥ 40kg/m^2 (also referred to as severe, extreme, or morbid obesity)

Risks

Maternal

- Gestational diabetes
- Hypertension – gestational hypertension and pre-eclampsia
- Vitamin D deficiency
- Induction of labour – spontaneous and iatrogenic
- Increased risk of failed induction of labour
- Prolonged labour – failure to progress, poor contractions, dysfunctional labour
- Problems with analgesia – failed epidurals
- Operative vaginal birth
- Caesarean section – elective and emergency and risks of the caesarean section
    - also, technically more difficult
- Failed vaginal birth after caesarean section (VBAC)
- Postpartum haemorrhage
- Infections especially wound infections
- Thromboembolism in pregnancy
- Anaesthetic risks

Fetal

- Early pregnancy loss
- Congenital malformations
    - neural tube defects (NTDs)
    - cardiovascular issues
    - cleft palate
    - anorectal atresia
    - limb reduction anomalies
- Stillbirth
- Fetal growth restriction
- Macrosomia
    - shoulder dystocia and its complications
- There is a lower risk of gastroschisis

Management

Pre-pregnancy

- Advise on healthy eating and physical activity – advise on having minimal gestational weight gain
    - current methods have met with limited success due to late implementation and poor adherence
    - such interventions must commence prior to conception to improve both maternal and child health outcomes
    - new approaches are needed to increase adherence to lifestyle changes
- refer them for appropriate support – to the nutritionist and/or physiotherapist

Antenatal

- Emphasise the need for regular antenatal care preferably at a joint clinic with the dietician
- Recommend a low dose of Aspirin – 150mg daily at night
- Recommend performing baseline tests in the first trimester – urine PCR, serum creatinine, platelet count, liver function test and OGTT
- Discuss healthy eating and exercises at each visit
- Weigh at each visit – keep gestational weight gain < 9kg: this may reduce the risk of macrosomia
- Consider repeating OGTT at 34-36 weeks
- Monitor blood pressure – use an appropriately sized cuff

- Monitor fetal growth
    - in anyone with a BMI of ≥ 30kg/m^2, fundal height measurement is likely to be inaccurate
        - recommend a growth scan at 28 and 34 weeks as a minimum
- In women with BMI ≥ 50
    - offer CTG twice weekly from 38 weeks
    - recommend induction of labour at 40 weeks
- Discuss thromboprophylaxis
- Refer her for an anaesthetic appointment

Labour

- Recommend induction of labour as above
    - in others individualise the need for induction of labour
- Recommend an early anaesthetic review if this has not been done
- Anticipate shoulder dystocia – have an experienced person nearby at the time of birth
- Recommend active management of the third stage

Neonatal

- Monitor for neonatal hypoglycaemia

Recommended Reading

1. Hill B, Skouteris H, Teede HJ et al. Health in Preconception, Pregnancy and Postpartum Global Alliance: International Network Preconception Research Priorities for the Prevention of Maternal Obesity and Related Pregnancy and Long-Term Complications. *J. Clin. Med.* 2019 Dec 2; 8(12): 2119.
2. Lackovic M, Filimonovic D, Mihajlovic S et al. The Influence of Increased Prepregnancy Body Mass Index and Excessive Gestational Weight Gain on Pregnancy Course and Fetal and Maternal Perinatal Outcomes. *Healthcare (Basel)* 2020 Sep 24; 8(4): E362.
3. Hanson MA, McAuliffe FM, Louise Killeen S et al. New guidelines, position paper, and insights from the FIGO Pregnancy Obesity and Nutrition Initiative (PONI). *Int. J. Gynaecol. Obstet.* 2020 Sep; 151 Suppl 1: 1-3.
4. Ramsey PS and Schenken RS. Obesity in pregnancy: Complications and maternal management. UpToDate, Feb 2017.

5. Simon A, Pratt M, Hutton B et al. Guidelines for the management of pregnant women with obesity: A systematic review. *Obes. Rev.* 2020 Mar; 21(3).

CHAPTER FORTY-FOUR

OBSTETRIC CHOLESTASIS (INTRA HEPATIC CHOLESTASIS)

Typically, women with intrahepatic cholestasis (ICP) present in the second and third trimesters

- They present with pruritus especially of affecting palms and soles of the feet particularly at night and without any rash
- Pruritus may precede liver function test (LFT) abnormality
- They may have jaundice after onset of itching (10% of cases) with features of obstructive jaundice with some darkening of urine and pale stools
- If a woman is Hep C positive features of ICP may present earlier (around 28 weeks)

Diagnosis

- Pruritus with elevated bile acid (BA) level (> 10mmol/l) – there is no longer a need to perform a fasting test
- High ALT and AST occur 1-2 weeks before a rise in bile acid level
- It resolves after birth

Other laboratory findings include:

- Elevated liver enzymes and/or mild elevation of total bilirubin – rarely > 6mg/dl
- Moderate elevation of serum transferases (< 3-fold) especially ALT
- Normal or mildly elevated gamma-glutamyl transpeptidase (levels are much higher in other forms of cholestatic liver disease)

Always look for and exclude other cause of pruritus, of raised bile acids and of abnormal liver function tests

Severity

Mild: bile acid (BA) level 10-19.9μmol/L

Moderate: BA level 20-39μmol/L
Severe: BA level > 40μmol/L
Very high: BA > 100μmol/L

Risks

- Preeclampsia – with severe intrahepatic cholestasis (ICP). If it occurs it usually does so 2-4 weeks after the diagnosis of ICP, and proteinuria often precedes hypertension
- Gestational diabetes
- Preterm labour
    - spontaneous preterm birth (PTB). These women have an earlier onset of pruritus and the risk of preterm labour is related to the level of BA
    - iatrogenic PTB
- Meconium stained amniotic fluid; the risk is 19% compared to 11% in the normal population
    - it is related to increased colonic activity and not to hypoxaemia
- Stillbirth (SB)
    - risk of SB in women with BA > 40mmol/l is 1.5% compared to 0.5% in the control population
    - in a large study, risk of SB was:
        - 0.13% if BA was < 40mmol/L
        - 0.28% if BA was 40-99mmol/L
        - 3.44% if BA level was ≥ 100mmol/L
    - risk of SB is not related to serum ALT levels or severity of pruritus
    - risk of perinatal mortality increases with increasing gestational age. In a large epidemiological study, risk of PNM was:
        - 4.7/10000 at 36^0 - 36^6 weeks
        - 12.3/10000 at 37^0 - 37^6 weeks
        - 13.7 /10000 at 38^0 - 38^6 weeks
        - 18.3/10000 at 39^0 - 39^6 weeks
    - cause of the SB is unknown
        - it is not due to placental insufficiency
        - it is probably related to the sudden development of fetal arrhythmia or vaso-spasm of placental vessels
    - data suggest that the risk of SB is unaltered with use of Ursodeoxycholic acid (UDCA) to lower bile acid levels

- Fetal intracranial haemorrhage (due to low Vitamin K)
- Neonatal respiratory distress syndrome (RDS) associated with bile in lungs and iatrogenic prematurity
    - BA affects the alveoli enzyme function which reduces surfactant levels

Management
Monitoring

- Monitor serum BA and LFTs weekly
- Recommend coagulation studies especially prior to induction of labour
- No method of antenatal monitoring will predict or prevent SB
    - even though the mechanism of SB is thought to be a sudden event most clinicians still offer a cardiotocography to detect acute compromise
- **Medications to treat symptoms mostly**
    - Cholestyramine, 4mg 2-3 times a day to relieve pruritus
    - Chlorpheniramine 4mg or Promethazine 25mg at night may also help
    - Ursodeoxycholic acid (UDCA) is recommended in most guidelines – 250mg three times a day and up to 750mg three to four times a day
        - may relieve pruritus – shown to do so only marginally in "Pitches Trial"
        - may improve liver biochemical tests
        - has not been shown to reduce risk of poor perinatal outcome
    - Rifampicin can be added to UDCA if bile acids remain persistently high
    - Dexamethasone 12mg a day has been used in non-responsive cases
- Vitamin K is generally not used routinely
    - recommend it if prothrombin time is prolonged (10mg daily orally)

Labour and birth

- Recommend birth at:
    - 39-40 weeks if BA level remains < 40mmol/l
    - 38 weeks if BA is at 40-99mmol/l
    - 35-36 weeks if BA ≥ 100mmol/l

    - 37-38 weeks if BA > 40mmol/l with deteriorating liver enzymes or severe symptoms despite being on UDCA
- Recommend continuous fetal heart rate monitoring in labour
- Recommend screening for coagulation profile with prothrombin time, at time of first diagnosis and then prior to delivery

Postpartum

- Complete recovery is usually rapid after birth, usually within 48 hours
- Recommend a physician review at 6 weeks postpartum with repeat LFTs
    - if biochemical abnormality still persists, exclude chronic liver disease
- Recurrence rate in subsequent pregnancy is around 60%
    - it occurs at an earlier gestation and is more severe
- Increased risk of developing gall stones, liver and biliary tract cancer, diabetes, thyroid and Crohn's disease
- Contraception
    - Mirena is the first line contraceptive option
    - avoid oestrogen pills
    - if they wish to use OCP recommend a low dose oestrogen combined pill after LFTs return to normal

Recommended Reading

1. Walker KF, Chappell LC, Hague WM et al. Pharmacological interventions for treating intrahepatic cholestasis of pregnancy. *Cochrane Database Syst. Rev.* 2020 Jul 27; 7(7): CD000493.
2. Piechota J, Jelski W, Piechota J, et al. Intrahepatic Cholestasis in Pregnancy: Review of the Literature. *J. Clin. Med.* 2020 May 6;9(5):1361.
3. Smith DD, Rood KM, Smith DD et al. Intrahepatic Cholestasis of Pregnancy. *Clin. Obstet. Gynecol.* 2020 Mar; 63(1): 134-151.
4. Di Mascio D, Quist-Nelson J, Riegel M et al. Perinatal death by bile acid levels in intrahepatic cholestasis of pregnancy: a systematic review. *J. Matern. Fetal Neonatal Med.* 2019 Nov 19: 1-9.
5. Gantz A et al. Intrahepatic cholestasis of pregnancy: Relationships between bile acid levels and fetal complication rates. *Hepatology.* 2004; 40(2): 467.

6. Mitchell AL, Ovadia C, Syngelaki A et al. Re-evaluating diagnostic thresholds for intrahepatic cholestasis of pregnancy: case-control and cohort study. *BJOG.* 2021 Feb 15. doi: 10.1111/1471-0528.16669.
7. Metz TD, Pettker CM. Society for Maternal-Fetal Medicine Consult Series #53: Intrahepatic cholestasis of pregnancy: Replaces Consult #13, April 2011. Society for Maternal-Fetal Medicine (SMFM). Electronic address: pubs@smfm.org, Lee RH, Mara Greenberg, *Am. J. Obstet. Gynecol.* 2021 Feb; 224(2): B2-B9.
8. Chappell LC, Bell JL, Smith A et al. and PITCHES study group. Ursodeoxycholic acid versus placebo in women with intrahepatic cholestasis of pregnancy (PITCHES): a randomised controlled trial. *Lancet*. 2019 Sep 7; 394(10201): 849-860.
9. Ovadia C, Seed PT, Sklavounos A, et al. Association of adverse perinatal outcomes of intrahepatic cholestasis of pregnancy with biochemical markers: results of aggregate and individual patient data meta-analyses. *Lancet*. 2019 Mar 2; 393(10174): 899-909.

CHAPTER FORTY-FIVE

OVARIAN CYSTS IN PREGNANCY

Adnexal masses may be ovarian or nonovarian.

Non ovarian masses include pedunculated fibroids, hydrosalpinx or para-ovarian cysts.

Ovarian cysts are usually:

- Corpus luteal or theca lutein cysts – these are often noted at the first-trimester ultrasound. A "ring of fire", they are usually asymptomatic, simple and measure less than 5cm in diameter
    - 70 % resolve spontaneously by the early part of the second trimester
    - complex ovarian cysts measuring more than 5cm are most likely to persist
        - the majority are asymptomatic corpus luteal cysts and the woman may complain of pain if there is bleeding into the cyst
- Endometriomas
- Mature teratomas (dermoid)
- Cystadenomas
- About 10% of the complex ovarian cysts may be malignant
    - 50% are epithelial tumours
    - 30% are germ cell tumours
- In all cases one must exclude ectopic pregnancy

Clinical features

- Most women are asymptomatic and the cyst is diagnosed on a routine scan
- Some women present with pain if they're bleeding into the cyst or the cyst ruptures or undergoes torsion
- Tumour markers are often elevated during pregnancy and are of less value

Management

The majority of adnexal masses diagnosed in pregnancy are benign and will resolve spontaneously

- if asymptomatic and < 5cm diameter – recommend expectant management
    - consider ongoing surveillance in each trimester

  if asymptomatic and > 5cm diameter, recommend rescanning after 16 weeks gestation

Surgery is indicated if:

- Size is > 10cm
- Tumours contain solid, cystic, papillary areas or are septate
    - recommend performing surgery at around 16-20 weeks gestation
    - in most cases surgery is laparoscopic
        - use mild inclination and a left lateral position in theatre
        - an open laparoscopy is preferable as opposed to the use of a Verres needle to obtain pneumoperitoneum

Recommended Reading

1. Goh W, Bohrer J and Zalud I. Management of the adnexal mass in pregnancy. *Curr. Opin. Obstet. Gynecol* 2014 Apr; 26(2): 49-53.
2. de Haan J, Verheecke M and Amant F. Management of ovarian cysts and cancer in pregnancy. *Facts Views Vis Obgyn.* 2015; 7(1): 25–31.
3. Mahomed K and Kumar S. Ovarian cyst in pregnancy. In: James D, Steer PJ, Weiner CP et al. Eds. *High risk pregnancy management options*. Fifth ed. Philadelphia: Elsevier; 2019. pp. 1101-1121.
4. Luque-Ramírez M, Ortiz-Flores AE, Nattero-Chávez L, Escobar-Morreale HF. A safety evaluation of current medications for adult women with the polycystic ovarian syndrome not pursuing pregnancy. *Expert Opin. Drug Saf.* 2020 Dec; 19(12): 1559-1576.
5. Liu YX, Zhang Y, Huang JF, Wang L. Meta-analysis comparing the safety of laparoscopic and open surgical approaches for suspected adnexal mass during the second trimester. *Int. J. Gynaecol. Obstet.* 2017 Mar; 136(3): 272-279.

CHAPTER FORTY-SIX

PARVOVIRUS INFECTION IN PREGNANCY

It is caused by parvovirus B19 mostly and commonly called slapped cheek syndrome or fifth disease.

- Transmission is by respiratory secretions, hand to mouth, blood products and trans placental
- Viraemia occurs 4-14 days after exposure
- Often affects children with fever, flu like symptoms and then a fine rash – occurs around day 15 by which time most are non-infectious
    - risk of infection in pregnancy is 3-4%
    - it is higher in teachers and childcare workers
        - risk from household contacts is around 50%
        - risk from exposure in a classroom is around 20 to 30%
- One attack confers lifelong immunity (40-60% are IgG positive)

Maternal/Fetal risks from infection

- Risk of transmission to fetus is 20-30%
    - if infected < 20 weeks, risks include:
        - fetal loss – 10%
        - non-immune hydrops – 3-10%
            - once hydrops resolves with treatment there are no long-term problems
        - fetal anaemia and progressive cardiac failure
    - if infected > 20 weeks, risks include:
        - fetal loss – 1-2%
        - hydrops is not a feature

Diagnosis

- Check maternal serology
    - if she is IgG positive and IgM negative, there is no concern
    - if she is IgG negative and IgM positive, this could mean a false positive or a recent infection
        - repeat the test in 2 weeks to detect IgG

            - if IgG is still negative (the initial test was false positive IgM), there is no concern
            - if IgG is now positive, treat it as a recent infection
    - if IgG and IgM are negative and a woman has had a recent exposure
        - repeat tests in 2 weeks
            - if she is IgG negative, there is no concern even if IgM is positive (false positive)
            - if she is IgG positive, treat it as a recent infection
    - if she's IgG and IgM positive – treat it as a recent infection
- A polymerase chain reaction (PCR) on the amniotic fluid may be performed – but it is not routinely offered

Management

Confirmed maternal infection < 20 weeks

- Advise that there is no risk of teratogenic effect but there is a risk of fetal loss (10%) or hydrops (3%)
    - recommend a scan 3-4 weeks after the onset of the infection and then 1-2 times weekly for about 12 weeks post infection
        - use MCA peak systolic velocity to diagnose fetal anaemia and scan for fetal hydrops, polyhydramnios, and cardiomegaly
            - if all are normal at 30 weeks, no further action is required and manage as normal
            - if there is fetal hydrops, consider a fetal blood transfusion after 22 weeks gestation
                - hydrops will resolve within 6 weeks of transfusion

Confirmed maternal infection > 20 weeks

- There is a small risk of fetal loss (1-2%), not associated with hydrops
    - otherwise reassure the woman and manage her as normal

Recommended Reading

1. Attwood LO, Holmes NE, Hui L. Identification and management of congenital parvovirus B19 infection. *Prenat. Diagn.* 2020 Aug 29. doi: 10.1002/pd.5819.

2. Palasanthiran P, Starr M, Jones C, editors. Management of perinatal infections. Sydney: Australasian Society for Infectious Diseases (ASID); 2014.
3. American College of Obstetricians and Gynecologists. Practice bulletin no. 151: Cytomegalovirus, parvovirus B19, varicella zoster, and toxoplasmosis in pregnancy. *Obstet. Gynecol.* 2015 Jun; 125(6): 1510-25. doi: 10.1097/01.AOG.0000466430.19823.53.
4. Crane J, Mundle W, Boucoiran I; Parvovirus B19 infection in pregnancy. *J. Obstet. Gynaecol. Can.* 2014 Dec; 36(12): 1107-1116.
5. Keighley CL, Skrzypek HJ, Wilson A et al. infection in pregnancy. *Med. J. Aust.* 2019 Aug; 211(3): 134-141.

CHAPTER FORTY-SEVEN

PLACENTA PRAEVIA

Predisposing factors:

- High parity
- Advancing maternal age
- Multiple pregnancy
- Previous caesarean sections
- Previous curettages
- Smoking
- Previous placenta praevia
- Submucous fibroids

Clinical presentation

- The majority have already been diagnosed at the 20-week morphology scan
- 70-80% will present with unprovoked painless vaginal bleeding
    - it may be provoked by coitus
- 10% of placenta praevia cases have coexisting abruption and thus have pain when they bleed
- The initial episode of bleeding is usually around 34 weeks
- There is often malpresentation and a high presenting part
- When there are multiple episodes of vaginal bleeding, it can affect fetal growth

Diagnosis

- It is diagnosed more frequently at a routine morphology scan – the placental edge is < 20mm from the internal os
    - request a transvaginal scan if in doubt with the transabdominal scan
    - at the morphology scan, as many as 7% are falsely negative for placenta praevia
- When the placenta is anterior, especially in a woman with a previous caesarean section (CS) exclude placenta accreta

  - risk of placenta accreta:
    - with placenta praevia it is 25% after 1 CS and 40% after 2 CSs
  - ultrasound combined with MRI has a greater accuracy in the diagnosis of placenta praevia with placenta accreta and has a low false positive rate
  - these women will usually be referred to a tertiary unit where options may include
    - prophylactic temporary abdominal aortic balloon (PTAAB) occlusion
    - placement of an occlusion balloon catheter in the internal iliac artery
    - prophylactic intraoperative uterine artery embolization
- If a scan shows a 2-vessel cord suspect the velamentous insertion of the cord

Risks

- Increased perinatal and maternal mortality
- Antepartum haemorrhage and/or placental abruption
- Fetal growth restriction if there has been repeated bleeding
- Major congenital malformations (twice as common in women with placenta praevia)
- Postpartum haemorrhage
- Anaesthetic problems
- Air embolism
- Placenta accreta in up to 15% of cases
- Puerperal sepsis

Management if she presents with bleeding

- If bleeding is slight to moderate and the woman is stable – allow prolongation of the pregnancy to as near term as possible
- This is possible even when the first episode of bleeding is quite heavy
- Monitor as an inpatient if the bleeding occurs after 30-32 weeks gestation
- Monitor haemoglobin and maintain haematocrit at > 30%
- Recommend a Betamethasone course if she presents with bleeding at 24-35 weeks
- Recommend Rhesus immunoglobulin in Rh negative women
- Use tocolysis with caution

- Request to have 2 units of cross matched blood available at all times

Management if asymptomatic

- She may bleed suddenly and heavily and the tradition has been to admit her to hospital from 34 weeks
- Outpatient management is also acceptable if:
    - bleeding has stopped for a week
    - she lives within 30 minutes of the hospital
    - there is an adult companion available 24 hours a day
    - she is reliable and will rest at home
    - she understands the risks

Placental location

Anterior placenta praevia is associated with increased adverse maternal and neonatal outcome.

Delivery considerations

- Recommend a single course of antenatal corticosteroid therapy between 34^{+0} and 35^{+6} weeks

Delivery is indicated if

- There is a persistent non-reassuring fetal heart trace
- There is a life threatening maternal haemorrhage
- There is significant bleeding recurring or persistent after 34 weeks
    - recommend delivery at 34^{+0} to 36^{+6} weeks in women who have a history of significant vaginal bleeding or if they have other associated risk factors for preterm delivery
    - recommend delivery at 36^{+0} to 37^{+0} weeks in the presence of risk factors
    - recommend delivery at 37^{0} to 37^{6} weeks gestation in the absence of risk factors

Mode of delivery

- Caesarean section
    - be aware that there may be placenta accreta
    - ensure pre-operative anaesthetic consultation
    - arrange for a cell saver
        - one may consider prophylactic intraoperative uterine artery embolization
    - a uterine incision may be modified depending on the placental site

        - consider the need to perform a vertical uterine incision
    - aim to find a placenta free space to enter the uterine cavity
    - if one has to go through the placenta – deliver the baby quickly, clamp the cord as soon as it is visible
    - they are at high risk of postpartum haemorrhage (PPH)
        - consider prophylactic Tranexamic acid (TXA) – it decreases blood loss and reduces the number of rescue uterotonics needed
        - consider the use of an intraoperative Bakri balloon if the bleeding becomes a concern
        - **see the PPH chapter on methods to prevent and manage PPH**
- Vaginal birth
    - a vaginal birth can be recommended in women where the placental edge is 11 to 20mm from the cervix
    - a vaginal birth may also be considered in carefully selected women where the placental edge is ≤ 10mm from the cervical os in an anterior placenta if:
        - the bleeding has not been of much concern
- Anaesthesia for CS:
    - if they are clinically stable, a regional anaesthesia is a safe option
    - a general anaesthesia is associated with a poorer neonatal outcome
- Recommend anti-D immunoglobulin for Rhesus negative women – use the Kleihauer-Betke test for dosage of immunoglobulin

Recommended Reading

1. Alfirevic Z, Bhide AG, Belfort MA et al. Placenta Praevia and Placenta Accreta: Diagnosis and Management. Green-top Guideline No. 27a. Royal College of Obstetricians and Gynaecologists *BJOG*. 2019 Jan; 126(1): e1-e48.
2. Jain V, Bos H, Bujold E. Guideline No. 402: Diagnosis and Management of Placenta Previa. *J. Obstet. Gynaecol. Can.* 2020 Jul;42(7):906-917.
3. Balachandar K, Melov SJ, Nayyar R. The risk of adverse maternal outcomes in cases of placenta praevia in an Australian population between 2007 and 2017. *Aust. N. Z. J. Obstet. Gynaecol.* 2020 Dec; 60(6): 890-895.

4. Ornaghi S, Vaglio Tessitore I, Vergani P. Pregnancy and Delivery Outcomes in Women with Persistent versus Resolved Low-Lying Placenta in the Late Third Trimester. *J. Ultrasound Med.* 2021 Mar 5. doi: 10.1002/jum.15687.
5. Guo P, Wu Y, Yuan X, Wan Z. Clinical diagnostic value and analysis of MRI combined with ultrasound in prenatal pernicious placenta previa with placenta accreta. *Ann. Palliat. Med.* 2021 Jun; 10(6): 6753-6759.
6. Huo F, Liang H, Feng Y. Prophylactic temporary abdominal aortic balloon occlusion for patients with pernicious placenta previa: a retrospective study. *BMC Anesthesiol.* 2021 Apr 29; 21(1): 134.
7. Levin G, Rottenstreich A, Ilan H et al. Predictors of adverse neonatal outcome in pregnancies complicated by placenta previa. *Placenta.* 2021 Jan 15; 104: 119-123.

CHAPTER FORTY-EIGHT

POLYHYDRAMNIOS

This is defined as amniotic fluid index (AFI) of ≥ 24 cm or a single deepest pocket (SDP) of ≥ 8 cm.

- Up to 30% of pregnancies with severe polyhydramnios (AFI ≥ 35 cm) have a major congenital anomaly

Aetiology

- Idiopathic polyhydramnios accounts for 50% to 60% of cases
- Congenital anomalies 8–45%
    - central nervous system (28%)
    - cardiac (22%)
    - gastrointestinal (14%)
    - others include thoracic, craniofacial, skeletal, renal and ventral wall anomalies
- Fetal aneuploidy – trisomy 21, 18 and 13
- Duodenal atresia and tracheo-oesophageal fistula
- Maternal diabetes (5-26%) – usually associated with poor control
- Multiple pregnancy
- Fetal anaemia including Rhesus isoimmunisation
- Congenital viral infections – CMV and Parvo virus infection
- Maternal substance abuse and smoking
- Placental abnormality such as angiomas

Risks

There is an increased risk of:

- Preterm premature rupture of membranes and preterm birth
- Malpresentation
- Cord complications – cord prolapse
- Caesarean section
- Increased perinatal mortality

Investigations

- If she is red cell antibody positive
  - assess for fetal anaemia
- If she is negative
  - test for cytomegalovirus and parvovirus infection
  - screen for haemoglobinopathies
  - exclude maternal diabetes
- Consider cordocentesis
  - for diagnosis and treatment of fetal anaemia
  - for karyotyping

Management

If she is asymptomatic – recommend expectant care as many will resolve spontaneously.

If she is symptomatic

- recommend serial amnioreductions
  - it is usually required if there is a fetal infection or if there is twin-twin transfusion
    - remove 1-5L at a time
    - aim to get SDP to < 8 cm
    - risks from the procedure include preterm labour, placental abruption, preterm rupture of membranes and intrauterine infection
- If < 32 weeks
  - recommend Indomethacin 25mg every 6 hours for 48 hours
    - a potential side effect of Indomethacin is premature closure of the fetal ductus arteriosus – the risk increases with increasing gestational age (50% risk at 32 weeks)
    - generally, it resolves within 24 hours after discontinuation of treatment
      - if polyhydramnios does not improve, recommend assessing for fetal wellbeing
- if > 32 weeks – individualise care

Delivery

- Recommend birth at 39 weeks gestation or later unless dictated by abnormal fetal test results or other pregnancy complications
- If she has an induction of labour, there is an increased risk of placental abruption and cord prolapse
  - consider transabdominal decompression first

- consider the use of a needle amniotomy or fetal scalp electrode to allow for the slow release of amniotic fluid

- Be aware of fetal malpresentation
- Be aware of postpartum haemorrhage

Recommended Reading

1. Sandlin AT, Chauhan SP and Magann EF. Clinical relevance of sonographically estimated amniotic fluid volume: polyhydramnios. *J. Ultrasound Med.* 2013; 32(5): 851-63.
2. Dashe JS, Pressman EK and Hibbard JU. Evaluation and management of polyhydramnios. Society for Maternal-Fetal Medicine (SMFM) Consult Series I #46.
3. Hamza A, Herr D, Solomayer EF and Meyberg-Solomayer G. Polyhydramnios: Causes, Diagnosis and Therapy. *Geburtshilfe Frauenheilkd.* 2013 Dec; 73(12): 1241–1246.

CHAPTER FORTY-NINE

POSTPARTUM HAEMORRHAGE

- Primary postpartum haemorrhage is bleeding within 24 hours of birth:
    - $\geq$ 500mL after vaginal birth
    - $\geq$ 1000mL after caesarean section
- Secondary PPH is any amount of bleeding occurring after this time up to 6 weeks

Risk factors for PPH

- Grand multiparity
- Multiple pregnancy
- Macrosomia
- Prolonged labour
- Placenta praevia/antepartum haemorrhage
- Polyhydramnios
- Placenta accreta
- Retained placenta
- General anaesthesia

PPH may occur in women without any identifiable clinical or historical risk factors.

Causes

- Atonic uterus 70%
- Retained placental tissue 10%
- Genital tract trauma 20%
- Coagulation defect

Prevention

- Anticipate
- Ensure pregnant women have an adequate haemoglobin level by term
- If she is a Jehovah's Witness and will not accept blood or blood products ensure a clear health directive is in place

At birth

- Ensure there is a 16g IV cannula in situ
- Send blood for group and hold or cross match 2 units depending on the severity of the risk factor
- recommend active management of the third stage: (reduces risk of primary PPH of > 1000ml and of maternal Hb less than 90g/l).
    - for women delivering vaginally
        - recommend Syntocinon 10IU intramuscularly with the birth of the anterior shoulder or immediately after the birth of the baby and before the cord is clamped
        - recommend a Syntocinon infusion – 40iu in 500ml at 10IU per hour
            - neither Carboprost (Prostaglandin F2a analogue) nor Misoprostol are better than Syntocinon in the prevention of PPH
        - a 0.5-1.0g intravenous injection of Tranexamic acid may be used in addition to the above for very high-risk cases (this has not been studied for vaginal births)
        - recommend delayed clamping of the cord
        - deliver the placenta by controlled cord traction with signs of placental separation
    - for women having a caesarean section:
        - recommend Syntocinon – 3IU intravenously slowly and repeat if required with or without an infusion as above
        - Carbetocin (100 micrograms given as an intravenous bolus over 1 minute) may be used and has been shown to prevent PPH in elective caesarean births
        - consider Tranexamic acid (0.5-1.0g intravenously) as it may reduce incidence of blood loss greater than 1000ml

Management of PPH

PPH with retained placenta – see the chapter on retained placenta

PPH after delivery of the placenta

- Recommend routine weight measurement of blood loss at birth
  - insert at least 2 (16-18 gauge) IV cannulas and an indwelling catheter
  - send blood for full blood count, chem 20 and coagulation profile (Rotem)
  - repeat 5 units of Syntocinon intravenously or 500mcg Ergometrine by slow intravenous injection
  - if not commenced, commence Syntocinon infusion 30IU in 500ml of either 0.9% sodium chloride or compound sodium lactate (Hartmann's solution) at 167ml/hr
- If she continues to bleed and her uterus is well contracted
  - exclude obvious bleeding from perineal injury and repair any lacerations
- If she is still bleeding
  - administer Misoprostol 800mcg via the rectum
  - give her 1g of Tranexamic acid intravenously over 10 minutes and a second dose 30 minutes later followed by an infusion of 1g over 8 hours
  - Prostaglandin F2 alpha (Carboprost) can also be used; draw up 5mg in a 20ml saline and inject it trans abdominally into the myometrium using a size 20 or 22G spinal needle
  - monitor pulse, respiratory rate and blood pressure recording every 15 minutes
- If she's still bleeding – prepare her for examination in theatre
- Whenever considering a planned procedure with a high risk of bleeding, arrange for possible intraoperative cell salvage
- Consider cell salvage also for emergency use in PPH associated with both caesarean section and vaginal delivery
- Replace blood loss/resuscitate and control bleeding – all often simultaneously:
  - Hartmann's 2L and Gelafusine 1.5L should be used until blood becomes available
  - X-match 4-6 units blood – if immediate transfusion is indicated, give group O, Rhesus D negative blood
  - administer 10ml of 10% Calcium gluconate for every 6 units of blood transfused

- ROTEM guided transfusion is helpful to guide coagulation correction:
  - it gives a quick result
  - it guides haemostatic treatment as it helps to diagnose the specific type of coagulopathic impairment
  - it reduces the need for blood products
- based on results, administer
  - rFVIIa
  - Cryoprecipitate and or fresh frozen plasma
  - platelets if the haemorrhage is ongoing and platelet count < 50,000/ml
- explore for cervical tears
- explore the uterine cavity for retained placenta tissue – careful blunt curettage may be performed if completeness of the placenta is in doubt
- if the uterus is atonic inject Prostaglandin F2 alpha (Carboprost); dilute 5mg in 20ml of saline and inject it into the myometrium
- consider a uterine tamponade using a Bakri balloon
  - if the tamponade controls the bleeding – leave the balloon in for 4-6 hours to assess the efficacy before further surgical intervention
- if surgery is required proceed to stepwise uterine devascularisation
  - ligate one uterine artery
  - ligate both uterine arteries
  - ligate the internal iliac artery
  - use a B-lynch suture or a modified compression suture (Haymann) which does not require a hysterotomy
    - double vertical compression sutures have proved to be effective in treating PPH due to atony and placenta praevia
  - subtotal or total hysterectomy
  - embolization

Recommended Reading

1. Atallah F, Goffman D. Improving Healthcare Responses to Obstetric Hemorrhage: Strategies to Mitigate Risk. *Risk. Manag. Healthc. Policy*. 2020 Jan 21;13:35-42.

2. ACOG COMMITTEE OPINION, Number 794. Quantitative Blood Loss in Obstetric Hemorrhage: *Obstet Gynecol.* 2019 Dec;134(6): e150-e156.
3. Althabe F, Therrien MNS, Pingray V et al. Postpartum hemorrhage care bundles to improve adherence to guidelines: A WHO technical consultation. *Int. J. Gynaecol. Obstet*. 2020 Mar; 148(3): 290-299.
4. Arnold MJ, Keung JJ, McCarragher B. Interventional Radiology: Indications and Best Practices. *Am. Fam. Physician.* 2019 May 1;99(9): 547-556.
5. Phillips JM, van den Anker JN, Ahmadzia HK. Next Generation Medical Management of Postpartum Hemorrhage. *Curr. Pharm. Des*. 2019; 25(5): 549-555.
6. Evensen A, Anderson JM, Fontaine P. Postpartum Hemorrhage: Prevention and Treatment. *Am. Fam. Physician*. 2017 Apr 1; 95(7): 442-449.
7. Wattar BH, Tamblyn JA, Parry-Smith W et al. Management of obstetric postpartum hemorrhage: a national service evaluation of current practice in the UK. *Risk Manag. Healthc. Policy*. 2017 Jan 17.

CHAPTER FIFTY

PRELABOUR RUPTURE OF MEMBRANES

Definition

- It is classed as term prelabour rupture of membranes (PROM) if the membranes rupture after ≥ 37 weeks and preterm PROM (or PPROM) if it occurs < 37 weeks

Incidence – 10% of all pregnancies

- 8% at term; 60% will labour spontaneously within 24 hours and > 90% within 48 hours
- 2-3% preterm
- < 1% mid-trimester

Risks from PROM

Maternal

- Chorioamnionitis (5-10%); the risk increases with duration as well as with number of digital vaginal examinations
- Placental abruption (associated with 4-7% of preterm PROM)
- Risk associated with induction of labour (IOL)
- Retained placenta
- Endomyometritis (3-4%)

Neonatal/Fetal

- Preterm delivery and its problems
- Cord prolapse
- Neonatal sepsis
- Risk associated with oligohydramnios if prolonged PPROM
- Increased risk of malpresentations

Pre-pregnancy prevention

- If she's a smoker, advise that she cease cigarette smoking
- Pre-pregnancy vaginal culture in at risk women and appropriate treatment may be of some benefit

Management

- Confirm gestational age
- Avoid performing a digital vaginal examination
- Confirm membranes have ruptured
  - the history is usually quite clear – there is a gush of fluid followed by continuous leaking
  - on sterile speculum examination there will be pooling of liquor in the posterior fornix; if it's not visible ask the woman to cough, gently moving the presenting part and seeing if any liquor is visible
  - if still unsure test for amniotic fluid by using Amnisure or a similar test
  - an ultrasound may help – there may be evidence of reduced liquor volume
- Exclude cord prolapse
- Confirm presenting part
  - recommend a bed side scan
- Send a high vaginal swab for culture
- Send a low vaginal and perianal swab for Group B Streptococcus infection
- Exclude chorioamnionitis
  - maternal temperature above 38°C
  - maternal pulse > 100/min
  - fetal heart rate > 160/min
  - uterine tenderness
  - raised CRP or neutrophil leucocytosis in the absence of another obvious cause
- Exclude placental abruption
- Assess fetal wellbeing – CTG

Management options

1. Term Pre-labour Rupture of Membranes (PROM): after 37 weeks

Options

- Advise immediate aggressive management if there is evidence of chorioamnionitis
  - commence intravenous injection of 2g Ampicillin (or Amoxicillin) and then 1g every 4 hours, Gentamicin

    5mg/kg daily and Metronidazole 500mg every 12 hours until delivery and then continue oral Ampicillin and Metronidazole postpartum for another 3 days
  - if she's allergic to penicillin, recommend Clindamycin 600mg intravenously every 8 hours AND Gentamicin 5mg/kg intravenously daily
- If a woman is known to be a carrier of Group B Streptococcus infection commence parenteral antibiotics and offer induction of labour as soon as practicable
- If there is no evidence of infection active management is still the recommended approach:
  - induction of labour within 2 hours of admission and 6 hours of ROM results
    - less chorioamnionitis
    - less endometritis
    - less likely to require neonatal intensive care or special care baby unit admission
- Some women may decide to await to go into spontaneous labour:
  - 85% of these are likely to go into spontaneous labour within 24-48 hours
    - there is a significant increase in the risk of chorioamnionitis and endometritis in the mother with expectant management > 24 hours after PROM
  - if women choose to await the onset of labour at home
    - ensure CTG is normal
    - advise her to record her temperature every 4 hours
  - advise the woman to return to the hospital if:
    - she develops a fever (37.5°C or above)
    - the colour or odour of vaginal loss changes
    - there is any concern regarding fetal movements
    - she starts contracting
  - advise her not to bath but use a shower – bathing increases risk of chorioamnionitis
  - advise her not to wait for more than 72 hours as the risk of maternal and neonatal infection is high if not birthed by 96 hours

- Induce labour:
    - most studies, including the international Term PROM trial, have used Prostaglandin E2 but practice varies
        - it is useful if the cervix is very unfavourable
    - standard practice is to recommend a Syntocinon infusion for induction of labour
- Prophylactic antibiotics
    - commence antibiotics when membranes have been ruptured for ≥ 18 hours or with expectant management from onset of labour/commencement of induction of labour
        - give Benzylpenicillin 3g intravenously initially and then 1.8g every 4 hours until birth
        - if she is allergic to Penicillin, recommend Lincomycin (or Clindamycin) 600mg intravenously in 50-100ml over at least 20 minutes and then every 8 hours until birth
        - where there is a history of a delayed type (non-immediate) reaction to penicillins (i.e., no history of immediate reaction) characterised by a rash occurring several days after starting treatment, recommend Cephazolin 2g intravenously and then 1g every 8 hours
- Number of vaginal examinations
    - this is an independent predictor for sepsis; women who have had ≥ 7 vaginal examinations during labour are at an increased risk of infection

2. Preterm Pre-labour Rupture of Membranes (PPROM): before 37 weeks

- Avoid digital vaginal examination
- If there is clinical chorioamnionitis – initiate aggressive management as for term PROM (see above)
- If there is no evidence of clinical chorioamnionitis – offer expectant management
    - expectant management has been shown to be associated with better maternal and fetal outcome. Recommend:
        - corticosteroids if gestation is 23^0 to 34^6 weeks
        - prophylactic antibiotics for prevention of group B streptococcus (GBS) infection

            - Erythromycin 250mg orally every 6 hours for 10 days
    - inpatient
        - keep them in hospital for at least 24 hours
    - recommend outpatient management in selected cases and:
        - recommend they attend a day assessment unit twice weekly
        - monitor white cell count, C reactive protein and vaginal swab for culture
        - monitor temperature 4 hourly and advise they return to hospital if their temperature is 37.5C degrees or above or if they have any bleeding, contractions, abdominal pains or offensive smelling vaginal discharge
        - tell them to avoid vaginal intercourse
        - recommend they don't use baths or swim
        - advise them to notify hospital immediately if they have any concern with fetal movements
    - offer induction of labour at 37 weeks
- Cervical cerclage – it is unclear as to when to remove the suture if one is in place
    - generally, if gestation is < 23 weeks, recommend removing it due to the increased risk of maternal and neonatal sepsis
    - if gestation is 23 to 34 weeks, and if there are no contraindications such as preterm labour, non-reassuring fetal status or infections
        - it may be beneficial to leave the suture in and monitor the woman closely for any signs of infection
- Discuss the risk of preterm delivery, pulmonary hypoplasia, infection and prolonged NNU stay especially in the very preterm pregnancy

3. Preterm Pre-labour Rupture of Membranes < 24 weeks

- Management is based on the fact that currently 100% of babies born at less than 22 weeks gestation do not survive and that 97.5% of babies born between 22 and 23 weeks gestation do not survive
- Involve receiving neonatal/obstetric units in discussions where transfer may be required
- Involve a multidisciplinary team to guide parents whenever possible

- Discuss with the family
  - that it is difficult to give accurate short and long-term prognosis for the baby
  - that even with resuscitation and intensive care, many babies of very low gestational age may die after birth
  - the possibility that even if resuscitation is attempted and is successful, there may be future situations where withdrawal of life sustaining interventions is considered
    - generally, between 23 and 24^6 weeks, life sustaining treatment is guided by parents' wishes
- Aim to achieve in-utero transfer unless transfer puts the mother's life at risk
- If life sustaining interventions are to be initiated, and only if a specific gestational age is achieved (e.g., interventions only if gestation reaches 24 weeks), then arrange transfer to a neonatal intensive care unit just prior to 24^0 weeks
- Recommend Corticosteroids to women who are at risk of preterm birth
- Recommend Magnesium sulphate to women at risk of preterm birth at 23^0-30^0 weeks where birth is imminent, and life sustaining interventions are planned or may be a possibility

Newborn care

- If there are any signs of infection, perform a septic workup (FBC and blood culture) and commence antibiotics
- If there are no signs of infection but suspected or diagnosed chorioamnionitis – perform a septic workup and commence antibiotics
- If there are no signs of infection but a previous baby had EOGBSD, perform a septic workup and commence antibiotics if there are any maternal risk factors for EOGBSD such as:
  - ROM for > 18 hours prior to delivery
  - intrapartum or postpartum (within 24 hours) fever of > 38°C
  - GBS colonisation in the current pregnancy
  - GBS bacteriuria in the current pregnancy
- If gestational age is less than 35 weeks
  - and if the mother did not receive adequate intrapartum antibiotics (no antibiotics or antibiotics for less than 2 hours prior to delivery), send blood for FBC and blood culture and commence antibiotics

    - and if the mother received adequate intrapartum antibiotics, send blood for FBC only and monitor for infection
        - if there are any signs of infection commence a septic workup and antibiotics
- If gestational age is 35 weeks and above
    - and if the mother did not receive adequate intrapartum antibiotics, send blood for FBC and commence antibiotics (but only if there are any signs of infection)
    - and if she received adequate intrapartum antibiotics, observe her in hospital for 24-48 hours for signs of infection

Recommended Reading

1. American College of Obstetricians and Gynecologists' Committee on Practice Bulletins—Obstetrics. Prelabor Rupture of Membranes: ACOG Practice Bulletin, Number 217. *Obstet. Gynecol.* 2020 Mar; 135(3): e80-e97.
2. Thomson AJ; Royal College of Obstetricians and Gynaecologists. Care of Women Presenting with Suspected Preterm Prelabour Rupture of Membranes from 24(+0) Weeks of Gestation: Green-top Guideline. *BJOG*. 2019 Aug; 126(9): e152-e166.
3. Tsakiridis I, Mamopoulos A, Chalkia-Prapa EM et al. Preterm Premature Rupture of Membranes: A Review of 3 National Guidelines. *Obstet. Gynecol. Surv.* 2018 Jun; 73(6): 368-375.
4. Schmitz T, Sentilhes L, Lorthe E, Preterm premature rupture of the membranes: Guidelines for clinical practice from the French College of Gynaecologists and Obstetricians (CNGOF). *Eur. J. Obstet. Gynecol. Reprod. Biol.* 2019 May; 236: 1-6.
5. Thumm B, Walsh G, Heyborne KD. Diagnosis of rupture of membranes: AmniSure, clinical assessment, and the Food and Drug Administration warning. *Am. J. Obstet. Gynecol MFM.* 2020 Nov; 2(4): 100200.
6. Dotters-Katz S. Antibiotics for Prophylaxis in the Setting of Preterm Prelabor Rupture of Membranes. *Obstet. Gynecol. Clin. North Am.* 2020 Dec; 47(4): 595-603.
7. Conde-Agudelo A, Romero R, Jung EJ, Garcia Sánchez ÁJ. Management of clinical chorioamnionitis: an evidence-based approach. *Am. J. Obstet. Gynecol.* 2020 Dec; 223(6): 848-869.

CHAPTER FIFTY-ONE

PRETERM LABOUR

Occurs in 6-8% of all deliveries and accounts for 70% of PNM and 50% of long-term neurological morbidity.

- 40% are spontaneous preterm labour
- 35% follow PPROM
- 25% are iatrogenic
- Up to 50% of women presenting with threatened preterm labour (TPTL) do not require any treatment and are probably not in labour

Causes

- Placental bleeding
- PIH
- PPROM
- Chorioamnionitis
- Cervical incompetence
- Bacteriuria
- Maternal cigarette smoking and substance abuse
- Pyrexia from any cause
- Excessive uterine enlargement – polyhydramnios, multiple pregnancy
- Uterine distortion – fibroids, uterine abnormality

Risks

Maternal

- These are related to the use of drugs to stop PTL or are associated with either the cause or result of the birthing process

Fetus

- There is increased perinatal morbidity and mortality due to:
    - a compromised fetus precipitating the PTL (FGR, congenital anomaly or infection)
    - risks of prematurity – hypoxia, birth trauma, RDS, NEC, intracranial haemorrhage and sepsis

Prevention

General

- These include making changes related to lifestyle, work and workload, physical exertion, nutrition, smoking, and substance abuse

Antenatal screening to identify women at risk:

- Previous history of PTB – with one previous preterm birth there is 15-20% risk of another, with 2, the risk is > 40%
- Low pre-pregnancy BMI
- Infection
    - screen at risk women at 24-26 weeks
        - treat bacterial vaginosis if it is present
        - if she has candidiasis, recommend treatment
- Cervical length (CL) screening – recommended a trans vaginal (TV) scan
    - short CL is defined as CL < 25mm length. Funnelling appears to be of no consequence.
    - recommend measuring transabdominal CL routinely at morphology scan at 20 weeks
        - recommend TV CL for those with abdominal CL < 35mm at morphology scan
        - recommend TV CL at 16 weeks gestation in all women with a previous singleton or twin preterm birth
            - if TV CL is > 30mm, request TV CL every 2 weeks between 16 and 24 weeks
            - if TV CL is 25-29mm, request TV CL weekly up to 24 weeks
- There is some evidence that screening at risk women for fetal fibronectin may be of use in identifying women likely to go into preterm labour

Prevention for PTL: Options include Progesterone, cervical cerclage and Arabin pessary – current data on Arabin pessary do not support its use

- Singleton or multiple pregnancy with previous preterm birth < 34 weeks
    - if CL is ≥ 25mm or length is unknown
        - there is no benefit from Progesterone or cervical cerclage

- Singleton pregnancy without previous preterm birth
    - if CL is < 25mm
        - offer 200mg vaginal Progesterone daily until 34 weeks
- Singleton pregnancy with previous preterm birth < 34 weeks
    - if CL < 25mm
        - can recommend Progesterone or cervical cerclage
        - as cerclage is associated with greater risk of harm, recommend Progesterone as first line and repeat CL in 1-2 weeks
            - if CL remains unchanged continue Progesterone
            - if there is further shortening of the cervix, recommend cerclage and continue Progesterone
- Multiple pregnancy with previous preterm birth < 34 weeks
    - if CL < 25mm
        - recommend Progesterone as above
            - some data suggest it is of value only in women with CL < 15mm
        - cervical cerclage is not recommended

Management of threatened preterm labour
Initial assessment

- Assess gestational age
- Identify any predisposing factor(s)
- Assess fetal wellbeing using CTG (in early pregnancy it is normal to have reduced baseline variability and accelerations that do not go up to 15bpm)
- Recommend FBC, MSSU for culture
- Recommend a vaginal speculum examination
    - take a low vaginal/perianal and cervical swab
    - test for the presence of fetal fibronectin (fFN) (normally fFN is not present at 24-34 weeks):
        - traditionally a value of 50ng/ml was used as a cut-off point
        - recent studies show that fFN < 200ng/ml has almost zero risk of birth within 7 days and about 5% risk of birth < 34 weeks gestation
        - there is no need to give Steroids or admit her into hospital if there are no other concerns

        - if the level is > 200ng/ml, recommend steroid loading and transfer to a tertiary hospital depending on the level of the facility

- Keep special care nursery and paediatric staff informed
- Recommend a scan to estimate fetal weight and assess fetal breathing movements
- It may be useful to also measure TV CL

Make a decision to suppress or not to suppress labour

Generally, suppression is not advised if there is presence of:

- Advanced labour (≥ 5cm cervical dilatation)
- Active bleeding
- Any suspicion of placental abruption
- Severe pre-eclampsia
- Fetal compromise
- Severe fetal anomaly
- PROM with chorioamnionitis
- Gestational age > 34 weeks

Rescue cerclage

- Consider 'rescue' cervical cerclage for women between 16^{+0} and 27^{+6} weeks of pregnancy with a dilated cervix and/or exposed, unruptured membranes
    - discuss the risks of the procedure, particularly risk of rupturing membranes
    - the cerclage may prolong pregnancy by a few more weeks

Tocolytic drugs

- Use of tocolysis gives time for the steroids to have some effect as well safe transfer if required
- Recommend Nifedipine – 20mg orally stat and every half hour (3 doses) and then 20mg every 6 hours until contractions have ceased. There is no evidence for giving maintenance therapy for longer than 48 hours

Steroids

- There is clear evidence of a benefit in women with preterm labour between 24-34^6 weeks
- There may be some benefit between 35^0-35^6 weeks (number needed to treat [NNT] is 50)
    - give two doses of 11.4mg Betamethasone intramuscularly 24 hours apart. In some cases, one may give the second dose in 12 hours rather than 24 hours
    - if labour is successfully stopped or the woman re-presents in preterm labour later, recommend a repeat single dose of Betamethasone
    - caution should be exercised with repeat courses of steroids due to their possible harmful effects

Antibiotics

- These are not of any benefit if membranes are intact and should only be used to treat a specific cause for preterm such as a urinary tract infection
- Once she is in established labour, recommend antibiotics for prevention of EOGBD as usual; give her Penicillin 3g intravenously and then 1.8g four hourly during the course of labour. If she is allergic to Penicillin, use Clindamycin 900mg intravenously every 8 hours until delivery

Magnesium Sulphate ($MgSO_4$)

- Recommend $MgSO_4$ to women between 24^0-30^0 weeks gestation where birth is expected or planned within 24 hours; commence administration as close to four hours prior to birth as possible
    - administer 4gm intravenous bolus over 20 minutes with a maintenance dose of 1gm/hr for 24 hours or until birth

Management of labour

- Always include the Paediatrician and the special care nursery/neonatal unit prior to birth

If aiming for a vaginal delivery

- Recommend continuous electronic fetal heart rate monitoring
- Recommend antibiotics in established preterm labour to prevent EOGBD
- Avoid elective prophylactic episiotomy to improve the neonatal outcome

- Recommend a controlled slow delivery of the head, too rapid a delivery may cause a 'compression-decompression' injury with cerebral bleeding
- Recommend delayed cord clamping as it confers advantage to the newborn, reducing the need for transfusion for anaemia
- Collect paired cord blood samples
- Send the placenta fresh for histology and microbiology

Recommended Reading

1. McIntosh J, Feltovich H, Berghella B, Manuck T. For Society for Maternal-Fetal Medicine (SMFM); The role of routine cervical length screening in selected high- and low-risk women for preterm birth prevention. *Consult Series* 2016: 40.
2. Romero R, Conde-Agudelo A, Da Fonseca E, O'Brien JM, Cetingoz E, Creasy JW, Hassan SS, Nicolaides KH. Vaginal progesterone for preventing preterm birth and adverse perinatal outcomes in singleton gestations with a short cervix: a meta-analysis of individual patient data. *Am. J. Obstet. Gynecol.* 2018; 218 (2): 161-80.
3. Conde-Agudelo A, Romero R, Da Fonseca E, O'Brien JM, Cetingoz E, Creasy, GW, Hassan SS, Erez O et al. Vaginal progesterone is as effective as cervical cerclage to prevent preterm birth in women with a singleton gestation, previous spontaneous preterm birth, and a short cervix: updated indirect comparison meta-analysis. *American Journal of Obstetrics & Gynecology* 2018.
4. Abbott DS, Radford SK, Seed PT et al. Evaluation of a quantitative fetal fibronectin test for spontaneous preterm birth in symptomatic women. *Amer. J. Obstet. Gynecol.* 2013; 208(2): 122. e1-6.
5. Hezelgrave NL, Shennan AH. Quantitative fetal fibronectin to predict spontaneous preterm birth: a review. *Womens Health* 2016; 12(1): 121–128.
6. Berghella V, Saccone G. Fetal fibronectin testing for prevention of preterm birth in singleton pregnancies with threatened preterm labor: a systematic review and meta-analysis of randomized controlled trials. *Amer. J. Obstet. Gynecol.* 2016; 215(4): 431-8.

CHAPTER FIFTY-TWO

RECURRENT MISCARRIAGES

This is defined as 3 or more pregnancy losses (some say 2 or more clinical confirmed pregnancy losses)

- Primary – multiple pregnancy losses with no live birth
- Secondary – multiple pregnancy losses in a woman who has had a live birth previously

It is important to obtain a clear and consistent definition of miscarriages

- Whether these were biochemical or clinically recognised pregnancies
  - the risk of losing three clinical pregnancies is low compared to losing three biochemical pregnancies (0.3% vs 22%)

Risk factors

A definitive cause is found in < 50% of women

- Age – both maternal > 35 years and paternal > 40 years
- Previous miscarriage (up to 40% after 3 miscarriages)
- Obesity
- Genetic factors
  - these are present in 10-15% of clinical pregnancy losses
  - 3-5% of partners have a chromosomal abnormality
  - generally, recommend karyotyping on products of conception after the third pregnancy loss
    - most sporadic miscarriages result from random numeric chromosomal errors involving 45 or 47 chromosomes
- Anatomical factors (10-15%)
  - congenital uterine malformations
    - these are present in 4.3% of the general population versus 12.6% of women with recurrent miscarriage (RM)

        - the commonest abnormality is a septate uterus; others include a unicornuate uterus, uterine didelphys, and bicornuate and arcuate uteri
        - these are usually associated with second trimester losses
    - acquired uterine abnormalities include adhesions, polyps, fibroids and intrauterine adhesions and uterine abnormality associated with Diethyl stilboestrol (DES) exposure in utero
- Cervical incompetence
    - clinical history may be useful to guide diagnosis (preceded by SROM and painless cervical dilatation; usually these are mid-trimester. It is not a cause for recurrent early miscarriages
- Infection
    - associated with sporadic miscarriage but probably not with recurrent miscarriages
        - these include Mycoplasma Hominis, Chlamydia, Listeria Monocytogenes, Ureaplasma Urealyticum and TORCH group
            - if positive for Mycoplasma or Ureaplasma – some suggest treating with Doxycycline 100mg twice daily for 14 days
- Endocrine factors may contribute to 8-12% of RM
    - luteal phase defect – serum Progesterone is < 10ng/ml in the luteal phase. Recommend vaginal Progesterone as soon as the pregnancy is diagnosed and continue up to 14 weeks gestation
        - Polycystic ovary syndrome (PCOS) – 30-50% of women with recurrent miscarriage have PCOS diagnosed on a U/S scan. If they hyper-secrete LH, they may be at increased risk of infertility and recurrent miscarriage
    - thyroid disease – untreated hypothyroidism or subclinical hypothyroidism may be associated with RM. Hyperthyroidism is not associated with RM
        - euthyroid women with thyroid antibodies have a higher risk of RM
    - poorly controlled diabetes
    - hyperprolactinaemia

- Thrombophilia
    - association between RM and inherited thrombophilia is weak
    - antiphospholipid syndrome (APLS) is present in 5-20% of women with RM – they have antiphospholipid antibodies (lupus anticoagulant. anticardiolipin antibody, beta 2 glycoprotein and antibodies to phosphatidyl serine)
        - ANA – 10-15% of normal women are positive – there's no relation to pregnancy outcome and it should not be tested
- Unexplained recurrent miscarriage
    - this is the case in over 50% of cases
    - informed and sympathetic counselling will give future pregnancy rates of up to 70%

Investigations

- Send products of conception for karyotyping
- Ultrasound scan
- Hysteroscopy
- Investigate for antiphospholipid syndrome
- TSH
- Factor V Leiden, prothrombin gene mutation and proteins deficiency

Treatment options

- Aspirin and Clexane
    - if she has APLS – recommend Aspirin and Clexane
        - initiate Clexane from the time of the positive pregnancy test until 6 weeks postpartum
        - Recommend a low dose of Aspirin (150mg at night) from prior to pregnancy until 34 weeks of gestation
            - there may be some benefit from the above also in women not meeting APL diagnosis criteria
    - if she has inherited thrombophilia
        - there is no benefit
- Genetic counselling – refer for counselling if she has an abnormal karyotype

- Surgical treatment
  - treat uterine abnormalities – particularly septate uteri and adhesions
  - uterine fibroids – recommended only if fibroids are submucous
- Progesterone
  - PROMISE trial of the use of Progesterone from positive pregnancy test to 12 weeks showed no benefit
  - another large randomized controlled trial (RCT) from the luteal phase to 28 weeks showed lower miscarriage and higher live births
  - some suggest Progesterone in the first trimester in all cases of idiopathic recurrent pregnancy losses
- Metformin – some have used this especially in women with high BMI
- Other options
  - psychological support in a dedicated pregnancy assessment clinic setting complemented with weekly ultrasound scanning has been shown to improve successful pregnancy rates
  - treat Bacterial Vaginosis (BV) or any other vaginal infection
  - introduce lifestyle changes – weight control, coffee, alcohol, smoking and cocaine use

Women with an unexplained recurrent miscarriage have an excellent prognosis for future pregnancy and so an optimistic approach can be encouraged.

Recommended Reading

1. Hennessy M, Dennehy R, Meaney S, A protocol for a systematic review of clinical practice guidelines for recurrent miscarriage. *HRB Open Res*. 2020 Oct 2; 3:12. doi: 10.12688/hrbopenres.13024.3
2. Papas RS, Kutteh WH. A new algorithm for the evaluation of recurrent pregnancy loss redefining unexplained miscarriage: review of current guidelines. *Curr. Opin. Obstet. Gynecol*. 2020 Oct; 32(5): 371-379.
3. Bender Atik R, Christiansen OB, Elson J et al. ESHRE guideline: recurrent pregnancy loss.

4. ESHRE Guideline Group on RPL. *Hum. Reprod. Open*. 2018 Apr 6; 2018(2): hoy004. doi: 10.1093.
5. Khalife D, Ghazeeri G, Kutteh W. Review of current guidelines for recurrent pregnancy loss: new strategies for optimal evaluation of women who may be superfertile. *Semin. Perinatol.* 2019 Mar; 43(2): 105-115.
6. Homer HA. Modern management of recurrent miscarriage. *Aust. N. Z. J. Obstet. Gynaecol*. 2019 Feb; 59(1): 36-44.

CHAPTER FIFTY-THREE

RED CELL ANTIGENS AND ANTIBODIES

Antibodies detected for the first time in the third trimester do not appear to cause haemolytic disease of the newborn (HDN).

Clinically significant antibodies include anti c, anti E. Fy^a and jk^a.

Lewis, I, and P blood groups

- IgM antibodies do not cross the placenta and are therefore not clinically significant

Kell

- Present in approximately 9% of Caucasians
- K, k, Ku, Js^b and Kp^b – can cause moderate to severe anaemia
- Kp^a, K^0 and Js^a rarely cause fetal anaemia
  - red blood cell production is increased to compensate for haemolysis
  - anti K antibodies also suppress erythropoiesis and thus cause earlier and more severe anaemia

Kidd

- Jk^a, Jk^b and JK^3 may cause mild anaemia

Duffy

- Fy^a can cause moderately severe anaemia
- FY^b can causes mild disease
  - all others have no clinical significance

MNS

- The MNS system contains the M, N, S, s, and U antigens, as well as 32 other rare antigens
- It is present in a small percentage of the general population
- Anti-S, anti-s, anti-U and anti-N may cause mild haemolysis

Management

- For clinically important antibodies, determine the maternal antibody level (use quantitative value)
- Recommend paternal phenotype testing for the target antigen (may avoid need for further testing and monitoring)
- In all cases continue to monitor antibody levels every 2-4 weeks depending on the gestational age and if the levels remain low
    - with all antigens, except anti K do not perform serial titres before 20 weeks
    - if titre is $\geq$ 1 in 16 commence monitoring using fetal middle cerebral artery doppler velocity
        - if MCA doppler velocity is > 1.5 MoM consider fetal invasive testing
            - treatment options include
                - therapeutic plasma exchange (TPE)
                - intravenous immune globulin (IVIG)
                - intrauterine transfusion
    - anti K antibody titre correlates poorly with the likelihood of fetal anaemia, and the severity of anaemia can change dramatically over the course of a single week
        - monitor for fetal anaemia in all these women with anti K antibodies
- Cell-free DNA testing of maternal blood can also determine fetal Kell, Rh(C), Rh(c), or Rh (E) status and will give a better predictor of HDN

Blood transfusion

- It is important to appreciate that if blood is required for these women it may be difficult to obtain blood due to difficulties in cross matching
- Request blood early so that a donor can be identified early and blood is available should fetal/maternal transfusion be required later
    - the mother may donate one to two units of RBCs during the second trimester
    - the mother's siblings can also be tested and requested to donate if required

Recommended Reading

1. RCOG green top guideline. The Management of Women with Red Cell Antibodies During Pregnancy. Guideline No. 65; RCOG 2014.
2. White, J, Qureshi, H, Massey, E, Needs, M et al. Guideline for blood grouping and red cell antibody testing in pregnancy. International Blood Group Reference Laboratory, NHS Blood and Transplant Unit. March 2016.
3. Tormey CA, Hendrickson JE. Transfusion-related red blood cell alloantibodies: induction and consequences. *Blood.* 2019 Apr 25; 133(17): 1821-1830.
4. Nwogu LC, Moise KJ, Klein KL et al. Successful management of severe red blood cell alloimmunization in pregnancy with a combination of therapeutic plasma exchange, intravenous immune globulin, and intrauterine transfusion. *Transfusion.* 2018 Mar; 58(3): 677-684.
5. Jator EK. Notorious anti-Jk3 in a pregnant woman. *Clin. Lab. Sci.* 2014 Spring; 27(2): 78-82.

CHAPTER FIFTY-FOUR

RETAINED PLACENTA

Definition

- This is when the placenta is not delivered within 30 minutes of birth, when the third stage is actively managed or within one hour when physiologically managed, without signs of postpartum haemorrhage (PPH) or maternal collapse

The placenta may be retained due to:

- Trapped / incarcerated placenta (separated but retained as cervix has closed)
- Adherent placenta
- Placenta accreta

Risk factors include

- Previous history of retained placenta (recurrence rate 10%)
- Advanced maternal age
- Previous caesarean section
- Previous dilatation and curettage
- Preterm birth
- Use of ergometrine
- Fetal growth restriction
- Uterine abnormality
- Vilamentous insertion of the cord (cord snaps and placenta gets retained)

Risks with retained placenta

- Postpartum haemorrhage
- Endomyometritis
- Uterine inversion

Management

- Ensure the woman has an empty bladder
- Avoid vigorous traction as this may lead to uterine inversion
- If she's bleeding
    - she must be taken to the theatre urgently for manual removal of placenta
- If she's not bleeding
    - try breast feeding or nipple stimulation
    - change her position
    - delaying intervention until at least 30 minutes have elapsed will lead to spontaneous delivery of the placenta in many cases
        - waiting as long as 60 minutes should only occur if the theatre will be able immediately if she starts bleeding
        - recommend Misoprostol 800mcg rectally
        - try a Carbetocin injection (100 micrograms given as an intravenous bolus over 1 minute)
        - umbilical vein injection of oxytocin solution may slightly reduce the need for manual removal
            - injection of Prostaglandin (such as dissolved Misoprostol) is being studied
            - the above strategies should not delay definitive treatment especially if the woman is bleeding
        - current evidence does not support the use of Nitro-glycerine
- **For second trimester retained placenta** – the risk of bleeding is low: it is safe to wait up to two hours from delivery as many will expel spontaneously
        - commence Syntocinon infusion – 30IU in 500ml saline
        - consider trying the above options as well

- **Manual removal of placenta**
    - it is performed in the theatre with good analgesia/anaesthesia
    - ensure a wide bore cannula has been inserted
    - avoid Ergometrine as it will make manual removal more difficult
    - if it's difficult to remove manually, try removing it with a sponge holding forceps to retract on an adherent portion

  - avoid sharp curettage as it increases the risk of perforation – if necessary use a large blunt curette
- If bleeding becomes a problem treat the woman as you would anyone with a **postpartum haemorrhage**

Recommended Reading

1. Belfort MA, Dildy III GA. Postpartum haemorrhage and other problems of the third stage. In: James DK, Steer PJ, Weiner CP, Gonik B, Crowther C, Robson SC (editors). *High risk pregnancy*. Fourth ed. Philadelphia: Elsevier; 2015. pp. 1283-1311.
2. Favilli A, Tosto V, Ceccobelli M et al. Risk factors for non-adherent retained placenta after vaginal delivery: a systematic review. *BMC Pregnancy Childbirth*. 2021 Mar 31; 21(1): 268.
3. Kumar N, Jahanfar S, Haas DM, Weeks AD. Umbilical vein injection for management of retained placenta. *Cochrane Database Syst Rev*. 2021 Mar 11; 3(3): CD001337.
4. Patrick HS, Mitra A, Rosen T et al. Pharmacologic intervention for the management of retained placenta: a systematic review and meta-analysis of randomized trials. *Am. J. Obstet. Gynecol*. 2020 Sep; 223(3): 447.e1-447.e19.
5. Denison FC, Carruthers KF, Hudson J et al. Nitroglycerin for treatment of retained placenta: A randomised, placebo-controlled, multicentre, double-blind trial in the UK. *PLoS Med*. 2019 Dec 30; 16(12): e1003001.

CHAPTER FIFTY-FIVE

RHESUS ISOIMMUNISATION

The major components are D, d, C, c, E, and e. The D antigen determines the Rhesus status. Absence of D indicates a Rh negative status.

- Approximately 15-17% of Caucasians, 5-7% of West Africans, 2% of Eurasians and less than 1% of indigenous Chinese are Rhesus negative
- About 60% of infants born to Rhesus negative mothers will be Rhesus positive
- Silent spontaneous feto-maternal haemorrhage occurs in 3% of women in the first trimester, 12% in the second and 45% in the third
- Risk of haemolytic disease of the newborn is greatest with anti D and anti c antibodies and coexistent anti c and anti E antibodies

Isoimmunisation depends on

- Amount of antigen (if it is < 0.1ml the risk of isoimmunisation is 3%, if it is 0.1-0.4ml the risk is 14% and if it is > 0.4ml risk is 22%)
- On the strength of the antigen (D is most potent)
- On the responsiveness of the mother (only two-thirds respond)
- On the ABO group of the mother and the fetus (if incompatible, red cells are destroyed before antibody formation takes place)

Prevention of isoimmunisation
Rhesus negative and Rh antibody negative woman
Recommend non-invasive prenatal testing (NIPT) to assess fetal blood type

- Overall diagnostic accuracy is well over 98%
- Avoids the unnecessary need to administer anti D immunoglobulin to women carrying an Rh negative child (occurs in 40% of Rh negative women)

Rhesus negative and Rh antibody negative – (NIPT is not available or not done)

- Recommend testing the Rhesus status of the baby's father – if he is Rhesus negative, treat the pregnancy as normal and there is no need to offer anti D immunoglobulin
- If the partner is Rh Positive or his status is unknown, assume he is Rhesus positive
    - recommend 625 IU Rh(D) immunoglobulin at 28 and 34 weeks gestation

Immuno-prophylaxis after sensitising events in women with no preformed antibodies

- First trimester – up to and including 12 weeks (dose of Rh immunoglobulin is 250IU)
    - miscarriage
    - threatened miscarriage with significant pain
        - if they continue to bleed intermittently repeat the dose every 6 weeks
    - termination of pregnancy
    - ectopic pregnancy
    - chorionic villus sampling
- Beyond the first trimester – after 12 weeks (dose of Rh immunoglobulin is 625IU)
    - chorionic villus sampling
    - amniocentesis
    - cordocentesis
    - abdominal trauma
    - each incidence of APH
    - external cephalic version

Repeat the dose of immunoglobulin each time if the sensitising episode occurs after 2 weeks of previous antenatal immune-prophylaxis.

Women who decline prophylactic Rhesus immunoglobulin

- These include
    - women who object on religious grounds
    - women who will be sterilised after the birth
    - women who are certain that they will have no more children
    - women who are in a stable relationship with a partner who is Rh (D) negative

Management of isoimmunised women – Rh (D) negative and Rh (D) antibody positive

- If the titre is less than 1/16 or concentration is < 0.5mcg/ml (< 2.5iu/ml), recommend testing every 4 weeks until 28 weeks and then every 2 weeks. If levels remain low, continue expectant management with spontaneous labour at term
- If the titre is greater than 1 in 16 or rising or concentration is > 4iu/ml, refer her for tertiary centre assessment
    - o the aim is to detect fetal anaemia, treat in utero and plan the birth using:
        - MCA doppler velocity
        - cordocentesis
        - intrauterine transfusion

Delivery – women who are Rh (D) antibody negative

- Collect cord blood for fetal blood grouping and a direct Coombs' test
    - o If Rh (D) positive – recommend 625 IU Rh(D) immunoglobulin within 72 hours of birth, but before 10 days if missed
- Assess the magnitude of feto-maternal haemorrhage (FMH) – this may be by performing a Kleihauer-Betke test (it has a high false positive rate and thus is associated with unnecessary administration of Rh[D] immunoglobulin) or by flow cytometry (which is a more accurate but costly test)
- Some conditions are associated with a large FMH
    - o traumatic deliveries including caesarean section
    - o manual removal of the placenta
    - o stillbirths and fetal deaths
    - o abdominal trauma during the third trimester
    - o twin births
    - o unexplained fetal hydrops
- The standard dose of 625 IU is sufficient to protect against 6ml of fetal cells (12ml of whole blood). For a FMH of a greater size, offer an additional dose of immunoglobulin

ABO incompatibility

- It is a more common cause of neonatal jaundice
- Occurs in 15-20% of pregnancies
- The mother is group O and the baby is group A or group B
- As antibodies are present at birth, neonatal jaundice can occur with first pregnancy
- Babies develop neonatal jaundice within the first few days of birth

Recommended Reading

1. RCOG - Green-top Guideline No. 65. The Use of Anti-D Immunoglobulin for Rhesus D Prophylaxis 2014.
2. ACOG Practice Bulletin No. 192: Management of Alloimmunization During Pregnancy. American College of Obstetricians and Gynecologists' Committee on Practice Bulletins—Obstetrics. *Obstet. Gynecol.* 2018 Mar; 131(3): e82-e90.
3. Fung KFK, Eason E. No. 133-Prevention of Rh Alloimmunization. *J. Obstet. Gynaecol. Can.* 2018 Jan; 40(1): e1-e10.
4. Sperling JD, Dahlke JD, Sutton D et al. Prevention of RhD Alloimmunization: A Comparison of Four National Guidelines. *Am. J. Perinatol.* 2018 Jan; 35(2): 110-119.
5. Visser GHA, Di Renzo GC, Spitalnik SL. The continuing burden of Rh disease 50 years after the introduction of anti-Rh(D) immunoglobin prophylaxis: call to action; FIGO Committee Safe Motherhood and Newborn Health. *Am. J. Obstet. Gynecol.* 2019 Sep; 221(3): 227.e1-227.e4.
6. Prefumo F, Fichera A, Fratelli N, Sartori E. Fetal anemia: Diagnosis and management. *Best Pract. Res. Clin. Obstet. Gynaecol.* 2019 Jul; 58: 2-14.
7. Sperling JD, Dahlke JD, Sutton D et al. Prevention of RhD Alloimmunization: A Comparison of Four National Guidelines. *Am. J. Perinatol.* 2018 Jan; 35(2): 110-119.
8. Practice Bulletin No. 181: Prevention of Rh D Alloimmunization. *Obstet. Gynecol.* 2017 Aug; 130(2): e57-e70.

CHAPTER FIFTY-SIX

SHOULDER DYSTOCIA

Risk factors for shoulder dystocia (SD)

- Previous history of shoulder dystocia – recurrence rate is 7 times higher
- BMI > 35 kg/m^2
- Maternal diabetes – two- to four-fold increased risk
- Fetal macrosomia > 4.5kg (nearly 50% of SD occurs where birthweight is < 4000g)
- Post-term pregnancy
- Induction of labour
- Slow progress from 7cm to full dilatation
- Oxytocin augmentation
- Prolonged second stage, especially if followed by instrumental delivery

Prevention

- Some evidence suggests that larger infants are more likely to suffer a permanent, rather than transient, brachial plexus injury after shoulder dystocia
- Some evidence suggests universal third trimester screening to detect macrosomia (results in a slight decrease in the incidence of shoulder dystocia)
- Monitor fetal growth and estimate fetal weight to guide labour plan
- Ensure there is an experienced accoucheur present at the birth
- Induction of labour (IOL)
  - IOL for suspected macrosomia in a non-diabetic woman does not have any effect but does reduce the risk of SD and injury in a woman with diabetes and a macrosomic baby
- Recommend a caesarean section if EFW > 4.5kg in a diabetic and > 5kg in a non-diabetic woman.

Although EFW has often been used to define a macrosomic fetus other measures such as abdominal circumference (AC) to head circumference (HC) difference > 50mm may be more predictive of shoulder dystocia.

Management

- Recommend regular drills on how to manage SD at a departmental level
- Anticipate shoulder dystocia in at risk women
- Have a systematic approach
- Ensure a senior clinician is immediately available
- Suspect impending SD if:
    - the head is slow to extend and does not restitute
    - there is difficulty with delivery of the head and chin
    - you see fetal chin burrowing into the perineum (turtle sign)
- Generally it is diagnosed if normal axial traction fails to deliver the shoulders and head-to-body birth time exceeds 60 secs
- Utilise the HELPERR pneumonic
- **H**—call for help and clearly state the problem and assign a person to document clearly
- **E**—evaluate for episiotomy
- **L**—lay the woman flat, remove any pillows under her head and bring her close to the end of the bed. With one assistant on each side, hyperflex and abduct both the legs (McRoberts manoeuvre) and apply gentle traction to deliver the baby (up to 90% of cases will be resolved)
    - avoid downward traction as this increases the risk of brachial plexus injury; apply gentle axial traction at all times
    - avoid rotating the head
    - avoid fundal pressure (increases the risk of rupture and brachial plexus injury)
- **P**—pressure: request the assistant apply suprapubic pressure with the palm of their hand from behind the anterior shoulder (in the direction the baby is facing) in a latero-posterior direction. Apply gentle traction to reduce the fetal bisacromial diameter and rotate the anterior fetal shoulder into the wider oblique pelvic diameter (often the above two manoeuvres are performed at the same time)
- **E**—enter the pelvis
    - apply the Woods screw manoeuvre – place your fingers in the vagina and apply pressure to the anterior shoulder followed by pressure to the posterior shoulder to get it in an oblique position while the assistant is applying suprapubic pressure
    - use both hands, one to rotate the anterior shoulder in one direction and the other hand to rotate the posterior shoulder in the opposite direction
    - try the Rubin manoeuvre; apply pressure to the anterior shoulder toward the chest anteriorly (towards the fetal face).

If the fetal spine is on the maternal left, use the right hand and vice versa if the fetal spine is on the maternal right

- **R**—remove the posterior arm – enter the sacral hollow posteriorly, flex at the elbow and sweep the arm gently across the chest. Many do this first if McRoberts manoeuvre fails. If still not birthed, then try to deliver the posterior shoulder using the Menticoglou manoeuvre. Ask the assistant to gently flex the fetal head toward the anterior shoulder and place your right middle finger into the fetus's posterior axilla from the left side of the pelvis and your left middle finger into the posterior axilla from the right side of the pelvis. Use the two middle fingers in the axilla to pull the posterior shoulder downward along the curve of the sacrum. Once the shoulder has been brought down sufficiently, grasp the post shoulder and deliver it as above
    - posterior axilla sling traction (PAST): if the posterior arm and shoulder **cannot be delivered by any of the methods described** – use a large Foley catheter. Use the index finger and feed the catheter through the posterior axilla and retrieve it with the other index finger. Clamp the two ends of the sling and apply moderate traction to deliver the posterior shoulder. Use this as a last resort
- **R**—roll the woman to the 'all fours' position. This may increase pelvic diameters and with the assistance of gravity try to deliver the baby with gentle posterior downward traction

Other manoeuvres include

- Fracturing the humerus or clavicle
- The Zavanelli manoeuvre – with the use of tocolysis (boluses of 50-500mcg Salbutamol or 2 sprays of 400mcg sublingual Glyceryl Trinitrate 5 minutes apart), rotate the head to OA; flex and reintroduce into the vagina and perform an emergency caesarean section
- Symphysiotomy

Other points

- If there is a nuchal cord do not clamp it, if it's loose slide it over the head
- After birth, milk the cord a few times before clamping to minimise hypovolaemia
- Collect the paired cord blood for blood gases and base excess
- Anticipate PPH

Fetal morbidity

- Delivery of the body should occur within 4-5 minutes of delivery of the head. Fetal morbidity occurs from fractures of the humerus or clavicle, from brachial plexus injury and from hypoxic brain injury

Brachial plexus injury

- Brachial plexus injury and shoulder dystocia are complications that may occur at birth but are often not causally related

Maternal morbidity

- This is related to postpartum haemorrhage (11%) and third and fourth-degree perineal tears (3.8%)

Documentation:

- Record the timing of the delivery of the head and body and each of the manoeuvres performed
- Document the position of the fetal head at delivery
- Document the position of the anterior shoulder (left or right) particularly for medico legal purposes

Offer a debriefing at a convenient time soon after the birth.

Recommended Reading

1. Sentilhes L. Shoulder dystocia: guidelines for clinical practice from the French College of Gynecologists and Obstetricians (CNGOF). *Eur. J. Obstet. Gynecol. Reprod. Biol.* 2016 May; 203: 156-161.
2. Hill MG and Cohen WR. Shoulder dystocia: prediction and management. *Women's Health* (Lond). 2016; 12(2): 251-61.
3. Hill DA, Lense J and Roepcke F. Shoulder Dystocia: Managing an Obstetric Emergency. *Am. Fam. Physician.* 2020 Jul 15; 102(2): 84-90.
4. Moraitis AA, Shreeve N, Sovio U et al. Universal third-trimester ultrasonic screening using fetal macrosomia in the prediction of adverse perinatal outcome: A systematic review and meta-analysis of diagnostic test accuracy. *PLoS Med.* 2020 Oct 13; 17(10): e1003190.
5. Johnson GJ, Denning S, Clark SL, Davidson C. Pathophysiologic Origins of Brachial Plexus Injury. *Obstet. Gynecol.* 2020 Oct; 136(4): 725-730.

6. Robinson R, Walker KF, White VA et al. The test accuracy of antenatal ultrasound definitions of fetal macrosomia to predict birth injury: A systematic review. *Eur. J. Obstet. Gynecol. Reprod. Biol.* 2020 Mar; 246: 79-85.
7. Gilstrop M and Hoffman MK. An Update on the Acute Management of Shoulder Dystocia. *Clin. Obstet. Gynecol.* 2016 Dec; 59(4): 813-819.

CHAPTER FIFTY-SEVEN

SYPHILIS IN PREGNANCY

It is caused by Treponema pallidum and is acquired by sexual transmission.

Primary Syphilis

- The woman will develop a painless chancre (ulcers) around the genital tract with regional lymph node enlargement; chancres heal spontaneously within 4-6 weeks even if not treated

Secondary syphilis

- Occurs in 25% of untreated women
- It can occur up to 6 months after the primary infection
- They develop a fine maculopapular rash characteristically on the palms, soles, and mucous membranes
    - these often disappears within a few weeks
- They may get a fever
- They often have generalised lymph node enlargement
- They may get genital condylomata lata

Latent syphilis

- This is usually subclinical and diagnosed by a positive FTA test
- If untreated, up to 40% may progress to tertiary syphilis

Tertiary Syphilis

- The disease progresses gradually over years (occurring in about 30% of untreated cases)
- It affects the cardiovascular system (they may get aortitis)
- They can get neurosyphilis
- They can get gumma formation (nodules especially in the bones and skin)

Diagnosis

- Recommend the universal screening of all pregnant women
- High risk groups include:
    - certain ethnic groups
    - adolescents
    - women with a sexually transmitted infection in their current pregnancy
    - substance use in pregnancy
    - sexual contact with an infectious case
    - engaging in high risk sexual activity

Screening

- VDRL and RPR (venereal disease research laboratory and rapid plasma reagin) tests are used as screening tests for all women at around 10-12 weeks gestation
    - Monitor the titre if serology is positive
- Repeat at 26-28 weeks
- Test again at 34-36 weeks and at birth

Confirmatory tests

- FTA/TPPA (fluorescent treponemal antibody/Treponema pallidum particle agglutination)
- The RPR test is useful in determining disease activity and response to treatment while the TPPA confirms exposure to Treponema pallidum
- perform the test on cerebrospinal fluid for neurosyphilis

Point-of-care testing may be used to detect early syphilitic disease and provide same-day testing and treatment.

Treatment

- Recommend 1.8g intramuscular Benzathine Penicillin for a primary infection
    - if diagnosed in the third trimester recommend a second dose one week later
    - repeat RPR titre monthly (or at delivery) to confirm a downward trend
- Recommend 2.4mu Benzathine Penicillin 2.4mu intramuscularly weekly for 3 weeks for a latent infection or syphilis of indeterminate duration in the absence of tertiary syphilis
- Oral Cefixime for treatment of syphilis is showing great promise in pregnant women

  - with adequate treatment VDRL/RPR tests become non-reactive within 12-24 months

Neonatal congenital syphilis
Rates of transmission to a baby born to a woman with untreated syphilis is estimated to be:

- 70% for primary and secondary syphilis
- 40% for early latent syphilis
- 10% for late latent syphilis

Clinical features

- Maculopapular rash
- Hepatosplenomegaly
- Osteochondritis seen on X-ray
- Ascites
- Chorioretinitis

At birth

- Send the placenta and cord for histology and a PCR
- Request VDRL titre in mother and baby (use venepuncture or a heal prick – not cord blood)
- Swab any rash
- Repeat serology at 3, 6 and 12 months

Recommended Reading

1. WHO (2017) WHO Guideline on Syphilis Screening and Treatment for Pregnant Women. Geneva: World Health Organization.
2. Liew ZQ, Ly V, Olson-Chen C. An old disease on the rise: new approaches to syphilis in pregnancy. *Curr Opin. Obstet. Gynecol.* 2021 Apr 1; 33(2): 78-85.
3. Sanchez L, Harris T, Duford A, Duran N. Recognizing and limiting syphilis to prevent congenital syphilis. JAAPA. 2020 Aug; 33(8): 44-47.
4. Ricco J, Westby A. Syphilis: Far from Ancient History. *Am. Fam. Physician*. 2020 Jul 15; 102(2): 91-98.
5. Ghanem KG, Ram S, Rice PA. The Modern Epidemic of Syphilis. *N. Engl. J. Med.* 2020 Feb 27; 382(9): 845-854.
6. Jin J. Screening for Syphilis in Pregnant Women. *JAMA*. 2018 Sep 4; 320(9): 948.

CHAPTER FIFTY-EIGHT

THIRD- AND FOURTH-DEGREE PERINEAL TEARS (OASIS-OBSTETRIC ANAL SPHINCTER INJURIES)

They are seen in about 4-6% in primiparous and 2% in multiparous women.

Anatomy

- The anal canal (4cm in length) extends from the anal verge to the anorectal ring which is formed by the fusion of the internal anal sphincter, external anal sphincter and puborectalis muscle, and is palpable on digital rectal examination
- The internal anal sphincter is the circular smooth muscle of the bowel about 6-8mm above the anal margin

Third degree tear – Injury to the perineum involves the anal sphincter (external and internal anal sphincter)

- **3a:** less than 50% of the external anal sphincter (EAS) thickness is torn
- **3b**: more than 50% of the EAS thickness is torn
- **3c**: the external and internal anal sphincters (IAS) are torn

Fourth degree – Injury to the perineum involves the anal sphincter complex (EAS and IAS) and the rectal mucosa

Risk factors

- Asian and African Caribbean ethnicity
- Primiparity
- Birth weight > 4kg
- Persistent occipito-posterior position at delivery
- Shoulder dystocia
- Prolonged second stage of labour (longer than 1 hour)

- Midline episiotomy
- Water birth
- Instrumental vaginal delivery particularly with the use of forceps
    - most of these risk factors are unavoidable and are therefore not useful for preventing a 3rd or 4th degree tear

Prevention

- Head control – control delivery of the head using the left hand and not letting the mother push when the head is crowning, allowing uterine contraction to do the work (these two alone may decrease the incidence of OASIS by 50% to 70%)
- Perineal support using the right hand may also be useful but there is no clear evidence of this
- Recommend warm compresses to the perineum during the second stage of labour
- Recommend perineal massages during the last month of pregnancy and in the second stage of labour
- Upright standing or squatting may increase risk of OASIS
- Adopt a policy of "restricted" episiotomy (i.e., only if indicated), rather than "liberal" use (i.e., routine), for the prevention of obstetrical anal sphincter injuries
- Recommend an episiotomy with instrumental delivery in primigravid women (avoid the midline episiotomy). There is no difference between mediolateral and lateral (recommend starting at 6 o'clock at an angle of 60 degrees).

Diagnosis

- It is extremely important for long term morbidity to carefully examine the perineum (vaginal and rectal) after all vaginal births for anal sphincter injury
- Recommend systematic rectal examination for obstetrical anal sphincter injury prior to repair in all women with a tear that is more than superficial in depth
- Palpate with a "pill-rolling" motion using the index finger inserted in the anus and the thumb in the vagina. When the external sphincter tears, the ends retract and a cavity is often palpated along the course of the sphincter muscle
- The internal anal sphincter (IAS) appears pale (like raw white fish), is not very thick, and can be found 6 to 8mm above (cephalad to) the anal margin

Recommend training in digital rectal assessment for all staff as it can improve the detection of OASIS.

Management

- Avoid figure of eight sutures during the repair of the anal mucosa as they can cause ischaemia
- Suture material
    - there has been very little research carried out comparing different suture types used for sphincter repairs
    - some colorectal surgeons use non-absorbable sutures for repairs of anal sphincters (there is concern that such sutures may result in stitch abscesses or suture ends may cause discomfort requiring their removal)
- Repair anal mucosa
    - recommend an interrupted 3-0 Vicryl/Monocryl suture with the knots tied in the anal lumen or external to the anal canal.
- Repair the internal anal sphincter
    - look for thin pale pink tissue close to the anal mucosa (looks like fascia)
    - recommend end to end anastomosis using a delayed absorbable suture such as 3/0 PDS or 3/0 Monocryl
- Identify and repair the external anal sphincter (EAS)
    - as the EAS normally retracts, mobilize muscle fibres using Metzenbaum scissors for the dissection and grasp it with Allis forceps
    - recommend end to end anastomosis using 2-3 interrupted mattress stiches using 3/0 PDS or 3/0 Monocryl
    - end to end or overlap techniques have been used – one small study suggested overlap may be associated with less anal incontinence; most clinicians recommend end to end anastomosis
- After repair of the sphincters, reconstruct the perineal body to relieve pressure on the sphincter repair
- If the operating theatre is not immediately available, repair can be delayed for 8 to 12 hours with no detrimental effect

Problems related to OASIS

- Perineal pain from oedema, urinary retention and defaecation problems
- Dyspareunia and sexual dysfunction
- Abscess formation, wound breakdown and rectovaginal fistulae
- Anal incontinence - flatal incontinence, passive soiling, or incontinence of liquid or solid stool

Post-operative care

- Recommend single prophylactic intravenous antibiotics (2nd generation Cephalosporin). There is no evidence of any benefit from a longer duration of antibiotics
- Use NSAID suppositories to reduce swelling
- Prescribe a post-operative laxative such as Lactulose 20ml twice daily for up to 2 weeks with advice on diet and high fluid intake (it results in an earlier and less painful first bowel motion [no other benefit has been demonstrated])
- Avoid using constipating agents and bulking agents
- Document clearly the extent of the tears and the repair process
- Inform her about the nature of the injury and the need for careful follow-up
    - see her at 6 weeks
    - see her at 6 months and offer an endoanal ultrasound and if there is any defect refer to a colorectal surgeon for secondary sphincter repair
- Refer her for pelvic floor physiotherapy

Subsequent delivery

- Risk of recurrence in a subsequent pregnancy
    - the recurrence risk is higher with use of forceps and if the baby weighs > 3.5kg
    - the recurrence rate is higher in Asian women
    - the risk of recurrence is the same as the baseline risk at first delivery; both are around 5%
- Further vaginal delivery may worsen anal incontinence if it's already present
    - if she is asymptomatic there is no clear evidence as to the best mode of delivery
    - if she is symptomatic there is a risk of worsening symptoms; recommend an elective caesarean section

- there is no evidence to support the role of elective episiotomy in a subsequent pregnancy

Recommended Reading

1. Royal College of Obstetricians and Gynaecologists (RCOG). The management of third and fourth-degree perineal tears. Guideline No. 29. London: RCOG Press; June 2015.
2. Ness W. Obstetric anal sphincter injury: causes, effects and management. *Nursing Times* [online]; 2017; 113: 5, 28-32.
3. Wilson AN, Homer CSE. Third- and fourth-degree tears: A review of the current evidence for prevention and management. *Aust. N. Z. J. Obstet. Gynaecol.* 2020 Apr; 60(2): 175-182.
4. Sideris M, McCaughey T, Hanrahan JG et al. Risk of obstetric anal sphincter injuries (OASIS) and anal incontinence: A meta-analysis. *Eur. J. Obstet. Gynecol. Reprod. Biol.* 2020 Sep; 252: 303-312.
5. Harvey MA, Pierce M, Alter JE et al. Obstetrical Anal Sphincter Injuries (OASIS): Prevention, Recognition, and Repair. Society of Obstetricians and Gynaecologists of Canada. *J. Obstet. Gynaecol. Can.* 2015 Dec; 37(12): 1131-48.

CHAPTER FIFTY-NINE

THROMBOCYTOPAENIA IN PREGNANCY

Thrombocytopaenia occurs in 8-10% of all pregnancies.

Severity is classified as follows

- Mild: platelet count > 100,000
- Moderate: count 50,000-100,000
- Severe: count < 50,000

Mild thrombocytopaenia in pregnancy (120,000-150,000) can be seen especially in the third trimester in 10% of normal women.

Causes

- Gestational thrombocytopaenia (GT) – commonest and accounts for 75% of cases
- Immune thrombocytopaenia (ITP) – the platelet count is < 100,000 (3-5% of cases)
- Thrombotic thrombocytopaenic purpura
- Haemolytic uraemic syndrome
- Preeclampsia and HELLP syndrome (account for 20% of cases of low platelets in pregnancy)
- Viral infections
- Other causes include – drug induced (Penicillin, Aspirin, Indomethacin, anticonvulsants, Methyl Dopa, Heparin), lymphoma/leukaemia, folate deficiency, vitamin B12 deficiency, DIC (including Type 2 VWD), acute fatty liver, antiphospholipid syndrome and SLE

1. Gestational Thrombocytopaenia (GT) is the commonest

- This is a benign condition; the platelet count is normal early in pregnancy
- The highest frequency is in the late third trimester
- The platelet count is usually > 80,000
- There is no evidence of increased bleeding or bruising
- It is not associated with any risk to the baby

- It resolves spontaneously postpartum (may take up to 6 weeks)

Management

- Usually no treatment is required
- Monitor the platelet count every 4-6 weeks
- No diagnostic testing is necessary with count > 100,000
- If the platelet count is < 100,000 liaise with a haematologist and also refer to the anaesthetist
- Epidural is generally safe if the platelet count remains above 80,000
- Fetal risk is very low – if the maternal count is < 80,000
    - test cord blood at birth and neonatal blood on days 1 and 4 for platelet count
- Check the platelet count at 6 weeks to ensure it is back to normal
- It often recurs in subsequent pregnancies

2. Immune thrombocytopaenia (ITP)

- It is an autoimmune condition with antiplatelet autoantibodies (exclude SLE and APS and screen for Hep C)
    - it may be secondary to SLE or antiphospholipid syndrome
- Platelet count remains stable in many cases
- It may cause bruising (risk of bleeding increases with counts < 20,000)
- Exclude other causes of thrombocytopenia
- Antiplatelet antibodies cross the placenta and may cause fetal thrombocytopaenia in about 15% of cases (with risk of intracranial haemorrhage)

Management

- If the platelet count remains > 80,000, continue to monitor it every 4 weeks till term
- If the platelet count falls below 80,000, repeat the test every 2 weeks
- Liaise with the haematologist
- Recommend treatment if she is symptomatic or if the count drops to < 20,000 at any stage of the pregnancy or < 50,000 in late pregnancy:
    - recommend Prednisolone 1mg/kg per day for two weeks and taper it off gradually. It takes at least 4 days for an initial response with a peak response at 2-3 weeks (80% will respond)
        - if on steroids for > 2 weeks, recommend intravenous bolus 100mg Hydrocortisone 6-8 hourly in labour

    - prescribe intravenous immune globulin (IVIG) – 2g/kg over 2-5 days. Recommend administering it about a week prior to the scheduled delivery; 70% will respond within 2-5 days (effect lasts 1-4 weeks)
    - in some women both options may be required
    - Azathioprine
- Surgery is safe if the platelet count is > 50,000
- Epidural is safe if the platelet count is above 80,000
- During vaginal birth:
    - avoid FBS, FSE, vacuum and rotational forceps
- Avoid NSAIDs in pregnancy and postpartum
- Inform the paediatrician early
    - risk of thrombocytopaenia in infants is about 10 to 15%
    - check platelet count on day 1 and day 4
    - withhold administering Vitamin K until platelet count is known
    - there is poor correlation between maternal platelet count and neonatal platelet count in ITP
    - the risk of neonatal thrombocytopaenia is higher
        - if there is previous history of neonatal thrombocytopaenia
        - if she has had a splenectomy
        - if the platelet count was < 50,000 during pregnancy or < 100,000 at the time of delivery

3. Thrombotic thrombocytopaenic purpura (TTP) / Haemolytic Uraemic Syndrome (HUS)

- This is a life threatening rare condition
- There is microvascular platelet aggregation and subsequent blockage of small vessels causing tissue ischaemia
- It may be hereditary or acquired
    - acquired is more common and can present at any time in pregnancy

Clinical features

- Fever
- There may be neurological symptoms (can vary in severity)
- There may be microangiopathic haemolytic anaemia with raised reticulocytes and the LDH enzyme

- Platelet count is often 10,000-30,000
- There is renal dysfunction/failure

Diagnosis

- Presence of anaemia, thrombocytopaenia and schistocytes
- ADAMTS13 activity is < 10%
- LDH and unconjugated bilirubin levels are elevated
- There are impaired renal function tests
- Coagulation tests are usually normal

Management

- Multidisciplinary team with supportive treatment
- Recommend plasma exchange therapy (PEX) to remove the autoantibody to ADAMTS13
- Steroids may be required
- Platelet transfusion is usually contraindicated and should be reserved for treatment of severe bleeding
- Delivery does not guarantee remission
- It can recur in subsequent pregnancies
- Avoid oestrogen contraceptives

Recommended Reading

1. Mangla A, Hamad H. Thrombocytopenia in Pregnancy. 2020 Nov 9. *StatPearls* [Internet]. Treasure Island (FL): StatPearls Publishing; 2020 Jan–PMID: 31613485.
2. Fogerty AE. Thrombocytopenia in Pregnancy: Approach to Diagnosis and Management. *Semin Thromb Hemost.* 2020 Apr; 46(3): 256-263.
3. Baucom AM, Kuller JA, Dotters-Katz S. Immune Thrombocytopenic Purpura in Pregnancy. *Obstet. Gynecol. Surv.* 2019 Aug; 74(8): 490-496.
4. Eslick R, McLintock C. Managing ITP and thrombocytopenia in pregnancy. *Platelets*. 2020; 31(3): 300-306.
5. Committee on Practice Bulletins—Obstetrics. ACOG Practice Bulletin No. 207: Thrombocytopenia in Pregnancy. *Obstet. Gynecol.* 2019 Mar; 133(3): e181-e193.

CHAPTER SIXTY

TOXOPLASMOSIS INFECTION IN PREGNANCY

- It is often unrecognised as it may just present with flu like symptoms
- Infection is acquired from cats or foods contaminated with cat litter
- Transmission is transplacental (40-50% risk of vertical transmission especially if in early pregnancy)
    - with first trimester infection, there is a 10-15% risk of infection but if infected there is a high risk of fetal loss or severe neonatal infection
    - with second trimester infection, there is a 30-40% risk of infection and the disease is less severe and non-fatal
    - with third trimester infection, there is > 50% risk of fetal infection but neonatal effects are mild or may be asymptomatic at birth

Risks include:

- Miscarriage, preterm labour, symmetrical FGR and stillbirth
- Congenital infection can cause (chorioretinitis, intracerebral calcification, hydrocephalus/microcephaly)
    - 90% of newborns are normal at birth and symptoms develop later in life (blindness, deafness, intellectual impairment and epilepsy)

Diagnosis

- Check maternal serology
    - if both IgG and IgM are negative, it indicates an absence of infection
        - repeat test if symptomatic
    - if IgG is positive and IgM is negative, it suggests evidence of a past infection
        - no further action is required
    - if IgG is positive or negative but IgM is positive, it indicates a possible recent infection
        - repeat IgG and IgM and avidity

        - if there is a rising titre of either or low IgG avidity, it indicates a recent infection
        - if there is an inconsistent or low IgM or high avidity, it indicates a past infection and no action is required
- Polymerase chain reaction (PCR) on amniotic fluid is diagnostic

Management

- Some may choose termination of pregnancy (TOP)
- Consider antibiotic treatment:
    - $\leq$ 18 weeks gestation – Spiramycin to prevent vertical transmission until intrauterine diagnosis is confirmed
        - Spiramycin is safe (1-1.5g orally twice daily until birth reduces the risk of vertical transmission)
    - with a $\geq$ 18 weeks gestation with prenatal diagnosis (i.e., fetal infection confirmed by PCR) or if the maternal infection was acquired > 18 weeks (as fetal transmission rate is high): one can use drugs to reduce the severity of the disease
        - Pyrimethamine 50mg daily (teratogenic in early pregnancy) with 5mg Folic acid and Sulphadiazine 1g three times daily until birth
    - scan in 3-4 weeks after the onset of the infection and then 1-2 weekly for about 12 weeks post infection

- Treatment does not cure the affected fetus
- After birth, recommend an examination of the newborn by the neonatologist
    - if the blood or placenta is IgM positive or PCR positive – treat the infant with Pyrimethamine, Folic acid and Sulfadiazine for 12 months
    - monitor hearing, vision and neurodevelopment throughout infancy and childhood

Recommended Reading

1. Peyron F, L'ollivier C, Mandelbrot L et al. Maternal and Congenital Toxoplasmosis: Diagnosis and Treatment Recommendations of a French Multidisciplinary Working Group. *Pathogens*. 2019 Feb 18; 8(1): 24. doi: 10.3390/pathogens8010024.
2. Paquet C, Yudin MH. Toxoplasmosis in Pregnancy: Prevention, Screening, and Treatment. *J. Obstet. Gynaecol. Can.* 2018 Aug; 40(8): e687-e693. doi: 10.1016/j.jogc.2018.05.036.
3. Maldonado YA, Read JS; Diagnosis, Treatment, and Prevention of Congenital Toxoplasmosis in the United States. *Pediatrics.* 2017 Feb; 139(2): e20163860. doi: 10.1542/peds.2016-3860.
4. American College of Obstetricians and Gynecologists. Practice bulletin no. 151: Cytomegalovirus, parvovirus B19, varicella zoster, and toxoplasmosis in pregnancy. *Obstet Gynecol.* 2015 Jun; 125(6): 1510-25.

CHAPTER SIXTY-ONE

URINARY TRACT INFECTION IN PREGNANCY

1. Asymptomatic bacteriuria

- Occurs in about 3-4% of pregnant women
- It's usually seen in the first trimester and peaks at around 20-24 weeks
- It's diagnosed by a culture of > 10^5org/ml in the absence of any symptoms
    - the traditional belief was that if this was untreated, acute pyelonephritis developed in 20-40% of cases with the subsequent risk of preterm labour
    - recent data suggest the risk of symptomatic pyelonephritis may be lower but screening for and treatment of asymptomatic bacteriuria in pregnant women is still a recommendation that has a moderate net benefit in reducing perinatal complications
- Women with a past history of urinary tract infection (UTI) who have asymptomatic bacteriuria are at a higher risk of getting acute pyelonephritis

Predisposing factors include

- Previous history of UTIs
- Multiparity
- Multiple pregnancy
- Anatomical abnormalities
- Diabetes mellitus
- Advanced maternal age

Escherichia coli is responsible for 60 to 90% of cases.

Diagnosis

- It is usually diagnosed by a routine culture of mid-stream urine on the first antenatal visit

- In women with symptoms suggestive of infection, ward urine will show nitrites
- Urine sent for culture will identify the organism

Treatment – can use any:

- Nitrofurantoin 50-100mg four times daily for 5 days
    - avoid it in the third trimester (it may cause neonatal haemolytic anaemia)
- Cephalexin 500mg twice daily or Ampicillin 500mg orally four times daily for 7 days
- Trimethoprim – avoid in 1st trimester. Anti-folate action
    - in all cases repeat the urine culture to ensure adequate eradication of the organism
    - recommend suppressive therapy if bacteriuria is persistent – Cephalexin 250mg orally at bedtime or Nitrofurantoin 100mg daily for the duration of the pregnancy

2. Acute Pyelonephritis

- Occurs in about 2% of pregnancies but has a recurrence rate of nearly 25% in the same pregnancy
- More frequent in the second and third trimesters

Clinical features:

- They may present with fever, chills, abdominal pains, nausea and vomiting
- There is pyrexia and renal angle tenderness

Predisposing factors

- Previous history of UTIs
- Diabetes
- Renal calculi
- Polycystic kidneys or other congenital abnormality of the UT

Diagnosis

- Urine will show protein, leucocytes, red cells and nitrites
- Confirm by sending urine for a culture
- Perform a blood culture if pyrexial
- Check FBC and electrolytes

Complications

- Anaemia
- Acute respiratory distress syndrome
- Renal insufficiency and/or perinephric abscess
- Septicaemia
- Preterm labour – from infection but also as a result of the pyrexia

Treatment

- Admit her into hospital
- Recommend intravenous fluids as dehydration is common
- Lower her temperature rapidly if she is pyrexial
- Recommend analgesics for the pain (avoid NSAIDs)
- Recommend intravenous antibiotics until the woman is afebrile for 24 to 48 hours
    - Cephtriaxone 1g daily or
    - Ampicillin 2g six hourly with Gentamycin 5mg/kg daily if she is systemically ill
        - follow this by oral antibiotics (Cephalexin 500mg oral every 6 hours) for at least 14 days
- If she fails to improve within 48 hours exclude an obstruction/renal abscess – recommend a renal ultrasound scan
- Monitor renal function frequently if she is ill (acute kidney injury can happen)
- Recommend an ultrasound scan of the kidneys – exclude congenital abnormality, calculi or hydronephrosis
- Check her urine again after completion of the treatment to test for a cure

Non microbial treatments

- These include urinary alkalinization, lactobacillus probiotics and cranberry juice
    - none have been shown to be effective

3. Acute cystitis

- Occurs in about 1% of all pregnancies
- Women present with dysuria, urgency, frequency and low abdominal pain
- There is proteinuria, pyuria and/or haematuria

Predisposing factors are the same as those for acute pyelonephritis.

Diagnosis

- Mid-stream urine for culture
- Microscopy has a high false positive rate (presence of nitrites and leucocytes)

Treatment

- This is same as for asymptomatic bacteriuria
- Prevent a recurrence – encourage good fluid intake and double voiding to reduce residual urine
- Advise the cleaning of the perineum from front to back after defaecation
- Advise them to empty their bladder after sexual intercourse

Recurrent UTIs

- Occurs in 3-4% of pregnancies
- If 2 or more UTIs are confirmed, recommend a renal ultrasound scan to exclude renal calculi
- Recommend prophylactic antibiotics for the rest of the pregnancy – Cephalexin 250mg orally at night

Recommended Reading

1. Szweda H, Jóźwik M. Urinary tract infections during pregnancy - an updated overview. *Dev Period Med.* 2016; 20(4): 263-272.
2. Nicolle LE, Gupta K, Bradley SF et al. Clinical Practice Guideline for the Management of Asymptomatic Bacteriuria: 2019 Update by the Infectious Diseases Society of America. *Clin. Infect. Dis*. 2019 May 2; 68(10): 1611-1615
3. Betschart C, Albrich WC, Brandner S et al. Guideline of the Swiss Society of Gynaecology and Obstetrics (SSGO) on acute and recurrent urinary tract infections in women, including pregnancy. *Swiss Med. Wkly*. 2020 May 4; 150: w20236.
4. Maki DG. USPSTF recommends screening for asymptomatic bacteriuria in pregnant women but not nonpregnant adults. *Ann Intern Med.* 2020 Feb 18; 172(4): JC14
5. Smaill FM, Vazquez JC. Antibiotics for asymptomatic bacteriuria in pregnancy. *Cochrane Database Syst Rev.* 2019 Nov 25; 2019(11): CD000490.
6. Abou Heidar NF, Degheili JA, Yacoubian AA, Khauli RB. Management of urinary tract infection in women: A practical approach for everyday practice. *Urol. Ann.* 2019 Oct-Dec; 11(4): 339-346.

CHAPTER SIXTY-TWO

UTERINE INVERSION

Classification

- 1st degree (incomplete): inverted fundus extends beyond cervical os
- 2nd degree (incomplete): inverted fundus extends through cervical ring but remains within vagina
- 3rd degree (complete): inverted fundus extends down to introitus
- 4th degree (total): vagina also inverted

Risk factors

- Abnormal adherence of the placenta especially if a fundal implantation
- Congenital weakness of the uterine wall or cervix
- Weakening of the uterine wall at the placental implantation site
- Inappropriate fundal pressure – this may occur with poor management of the third stage
  - Crede's manoeuvre (squeezing the uterine fundus abdominally to deliver the placenta)
  - excessive cord traction before separation of the placenta or without counter-pressure upwards on the uterine fundus especially if the uterus is relaxed
- Uterine atony
- In > 50% of cases there is not an identifiable risk factor

Clinical features

- Severe lower abdominal pain in the third stage
- Postpartum haemorrhage
- The woman often develops shock that is out of proportion to the amount of blood loss
- On abdominal examination the fundus is not palpable in the correct anatomic position, and in women with a thin abdominal wall, you may feel a cuplike depression indicating the collapsed fundus
- On vaginal examination there is a soft, congested, bleeding mass

Management

- Avoid oxytocic drugs
- Establish secure intravenous access
- Do not attempt to deliver the placenta until the inversion is corrected
- Attempt immediate manual replacement
    - manual reposition (the Johnson manoeuvre) – with sterile gloves place a hand plus two-thirds of the forearm in the vagina and keeping fingers at the cervico-uterine junction and resting the fundus in the palm, lift the uterus above the level of the umbilicus. Keep the hand in the uterus until a firm contraction of the uterus is felt
        - the earlier this is done the better the success rate – it can be performed in the birth-suite if she has an epidural
        - to obtain a uterine relaxation may use Salbutamol – 50mcg boluses or Glyceryl Trinitrate spray 400 micrograms sublingually
            - once corrected hold the uterus in position for 3 to 5 minutes manually or by applying ringed forceps to the cervix to allow for countertraction
    - hydrostatic pressure (O'Sullivan technique) – exclude a uterine rupture before attempting this manoeuvre: set up saline infusion sets and hold the open end of the tubing in one hand. Replace the fundus in the vagina and place the right hand in the vagina and with the other hand block the introitus. Run the fluid fast and the increasing pressure in the vagina will gradually replace the fundus
    - Silastic cup technique – connect a 6cm silastic cup to a Y connector connected to a bag of warm saline, place the cup inside the vagina and infuse the fluid; the hydrostatic pressure generated will gradually restore the uterine position
    - if unsuccessful transfer her to the theatre:
        - abdominal approach – make a 5- 6 cm long incision in the posterior portion of the lower uterine wall through the cervical ring. Place clamps on the uterus at the level of the round ligaments and apply gentle upward traction progressively until the fundus is replaced. Close the hysterotomy in the usual fashion

  - vaginal approach – make a transverse incision in the anterior vaginal wall above the anterior cervical lip and into the anterior uterine wall. Apply upward pressure in the fundus to reposition the fundus. Close the defect in 2 layers
- The placenta can then be delivered once the inversion has been corrected
- Keep the uterus contracted using a Syntocinon infusion and rectal Misoprostol
- Recommend a prophylactic dose of antibiotics

Recommended Reading

1. Sunjaya AP, Dewi AK. Total Uterine Inversion Post-Partum: Case Report and Management Strategies. *J Family Reprod Health.* 2018 Dec; 12(4): 223-225.
2. Wendel MP, Shnaekel KL, Magann EF. Uterine Inversion: A Review of a Life-Threatening Obstetrical Emergency. *Obstet. Gynecol. Surv.* 2018 Jul; 73(7): 411-417.

CHAPTER SIXTY-THREE

UTERINE MALFORMATIONS IN PREGNANCY

- Seen in about 3-4 % of women
    - in up to 10% of women with recurrent miscarriages
    - in up to 20% in women with mid trimester loss

These include

- **Arcuate Uterus** – the uterus appears normal from the outside but has a very small (1cm or less) indentation, a concave dimple, protruding from the top of the uterine cavity into the endometrial cavity
    - generally, it causes no problems

- **Bicornuate Uterus (Uterus with two horns)** - most common form of a Müllerian anomaly. Uterus is shaped like a heart, with a deep indentation at the top. The baby has less space to grow than in a normally shaped uterus

- **Septate Uterus (Uterine septum or partition)** – the uterus appears normal from the outside, but it contains an internal septum that divides the uterine cavity into 2 smaller cavities. It is the most common uterine malformation
    - it can cause a miscarriage
    - it is associated with an increased risk of preterm birth and lower fetal survival rate

- **Didelphys Uterus (Double Uterus)** - both Müllerian ducts develop but fail to fuse, so the woman will have a "double uterus"

- **Unicornuate Uterus (One-sided uterus)** - only one side of the Müllerian duct forms. The uterus has a typical "banana shape" on imaging
    - a unicornuate uterus with a rudimentary horn does not require surgical correction

Problems in pregnancy are related to the size of the uterine cavity as well as its ability to distend.

In some cases, especially those with a bicornuate uterus there may be cervical incompetence.

Management in all cases:

- Recommend a TV cervical length measurement at 16 weeks and at 24 weeks
    - recommend vaginal Progesterone if cervical length is < 25mm
    - if she has had a previous pregnancy loss consider cervical cerclage
- Monitor growth and wellbeing at 28 and 32 weeks
- Exclude malpresentations
    - if all is normal await spontaneous labour
- If considering Mirena for contraception, place one in each of the two horns in a bicornuate uterus
- Recommend investigations postpartum to exclude renal tract abnormality if this has not been performed already

Recommended Reading

1. Ali S, Majid S, Niamat Ali M et al. Evaluation of etiology and pregnancy outcome in recurrent miscarriage patients. *Saudi J. Biol. Sci.* 2020 Oct; 27(10): 2809-2817.
2. Coelho Neto MA, Ludwin A, Petraglia F et al. Definitions, prevalence, clinical implications and treatment of T-shaped uterus: systematic review. *Ultrasound Obstet. Gynecol.* 2020 Sep 8. doi: 10.1002/uog.23108.
3. Pabuccu R, Pabuccu EG, Gomel V. Reproductive outcomes of patients with T-Shaped and septate uterus following metroplasty: an observational study. *Facts Views Vis. Obgyn.* 2020 Mar 27; 11(4): 317-321.

CHAPTER SIXTY-FOUR

VACUUM BIRTH

Contraindications

- Brow or face presentation that is not mento-anterior
- Operator inexperience
- Preterm infants < 34 weeks
- Fetal bleeding or bony condition

Prerequisites

- Obtain verbal consent
- Exclude cephalopelvic disproportion (CPD) – the presenting part should be at the level or below the ischial spines or the head should be less than two-fifths palpable above the brim with minimal or no caput and moulding
- Use an ultrasound scan to confirm fetal head position
- Empty the bladder unless the head is on the perineum
- Ensure adequate analgesia – recommend a pudendal block if she does not have an epidural. Occasionally local infiltration may be used but only if the head is on the perineum

If there is any doubt about possible CPD, perform the procedure in theatre as a "Trial of operative vaginal delivery".

Minimising the need for an operative vaginal birth

- Have a dedicated and continuous support person during labour
- Ensure effective uterine activity using Syntocinon augmentation
- Delay active pushing in women with an epidural
- Allow more time to push in nulliparous women with an epidural and no fetal heart rate concern
- Attempt manual head rotation into an occipito anterior position

Complications

Maternal

- Soft tissue trauma to birth canal and adjacent structures: uterus, cervix and vagina (these occur more following forceps than with vacuum births)
- Haematoma formation – immediate or delayed
- Bladder and urethral injuries leading to retention or fistula
- Rectal injury with subsequent faecal soiling, fistula
- Postpartum haemorrhage

Fetal

- Scalp injury (minor or severe) – bruising, abrasions, lacerations, palsies and fractures (these are more common with forceps than with a vacuum delivery)
- Cephalohematoma
- Subgaleal haematoma
- Intracranial haemorrhage and cerebral tears
- Neonatal jaundice and retinal haemorrhage (more common with vacuum births than with forceps)
- Brachial plexus injury

Procedure

Choice of cups

Soft plastic cups – These have a higher failure rate than rigid cups but are associated with less neonatal scalp injuries and are suitable for straightforward deliveries with no significant caput.

Rigid plastic cups – These may be preferable for delivery of occipito-posterior, transverse and difficult occipito-anterior positions.

- Although most people perform the vacuum with women in the lithotomy position, many lift out vacuum deliveries can be easily performed with women in the left lateral position
- Apply the cup on the flexion point - in a normally moulded fetal head the flexion point is about 3cm in front of the posterior fontanelle. The centre of the cup should rest as closely as possible to the flexion point. With a 50mm cup over the flexion point, the distance between the leading edge of the cup and the anterior fontanelle would be about 3cm
- Before inducing the vacuum ensure there is no vaginal or cervical tissue caught underneath the cup

- Apply traction in the line of the pelvic axis to promote flexion and synclitism
- Apply traction during a contraction and with the mother pushing
- Use one hand (right) to pull and use the index finger and thumb of the other hand on the edge of the cup and on the fetal head as counter-traction (this helps to confirm descent and also prevents the cup slipping off)
- Some data suggest that an episiotomy in all primiparous women may minimise the risk of OASIS
- Perform cord blood gases in all cases
- Recommend single dose prophylactic antibiotics
    - they are effective in reducing superficial and deep perineal wound infections or serious infectious complications

Abandon the procedure if

- There is no progress after the 2nd or 3rd pull or if the cup dislodges three times
- In selected cases one may use forceps to complete the birth
    - this is acceptable in certain circumstances and should not be labelled as a sequential use; for instance:
        - if after a failed vacuum, after reassessing, she is assessed as being a good candidate for forceps and the initial choice of vacuum was associated with poor maternal effort or an OP position
        - if a vacuum device fails to achieve suction or comes off with minimal traction and forceps are used
    - avoid a planned sequential use of instruments – this is associated with an increased risk of perinatal trauma

Documentation

- Careful documentation is required in the woman's chart both prior to performing the delivery as well as on completion
- Adopt
    - a checklist for preparation and performance of the procedure
    - a checklist for documentation
        - include details on:
            - examination findings
            - indication for operative delivery
            - anaesthesia used
            - personnel present

- instruments used
- time of the start and end of the procedure
- any complications

Odon device

- This has been developed by the World Health Organization and is currently being tested; it is made of a film-like polyethylene material that creates a sac filled with air that surrounds the entire head and enables extraction when traction is applied
- It is thought to be safer and easier to apply than the conventional vacuum
- Current data do not support any benefit over the conventional vacuum devices

Recommended Reading

1. Vacca A. *Handbook of vacuum extraction in obstetric practice.* Vacca Research Qld. 2nd edition 2003.
2. Vayssière C, Beucher G, Dupuis O et al. French College of Gynaecologists and Obstetricians. Instrumental delivery: clinical practice guidelines from the French College of Gynaecologists and Obstetricians. *Eur. J. Obstet. Gynecol. Reprod. Biol.* 2011 Nov; 159(1): 43-8.
3. Liabsuetrakul T, Choobun T, Peeyananjarassri K, Islam QM. Operative Vaginal Birth: ACOG Practice Bulletin Summary, Number 219. *Obstet. Gynecol.* 2020 Apr; 135(4): 982-984.
4. Antibiotic prophylaxis for operative vaginal delivery. *Cochrane Database Syst. Rev.* 2020 Mar 26; 3(3): CD004455.
5. Hobson S, Cassell K, Windrim R, Cargill Y No. 381 - Assisted Vaginal Birth. *J. Obstet. Gynaecol. Can.* 2019 Jun; 41(6): 870-882.

CHAPTER SIXTY-FIVE

VAGINAL BIRTH AFTER ONE PREVIOUS CAESAREAN SECTION (VBAC-1)

- Shared decision making is a collaborative, bidirectional method of communication
- Inform women of the risks, benefits, and prognosis but also elicit their values and negotiate competing priorities in the process of making a joint decision
- Multiple pregnancy is not a contraindication to a trial of vaginal birth after a caesarean section (CS)

Assess eligibility for a VBAC

- Exclude any contraindications
    - arising from the past pregnancy
        - a previous rupture
        - a previous upper segment CS (risk of rupture 2-9%)
        - a previous T incision
    - arising during the current pregnancy
        - placenta praevia
        - a clinically inadequate pelvis
        - other major uterine surgery
- Recommend a full discussion at the 20-week visit and again at 28 weeks to confirm and formalise her options

Success of a VBAC

- If a woman goes into spontaneous labour, her success rate is 70% after one previous CS
    - favourable factors for a vaginal birth include:
        - the reason for the previous CS not being a factor in the current pregnancy
        - a previous successful VBAC or a previous vaginal birth (success rate > 85%)
        - previous CS being for a multiple pregnancy or malpresentation

        - spontaneous onset of labour
        - her age being less than 30 years
        - BMI being less than 30
        - estimated fetal weight less than 4kg
    - unfavourable factors include:
        - previous failed instrumental birth
        - previous CS for dystocia or failure to progress
        - her age being 35 years or older
        - her BMI being greater than 30 or the estimated fetal weight being more than 4kg
        - induction of labour
        - previous preterm CS
        - gestational diabetes
        - pregnancy > 40 weeks

Risks associated with VBAC

- Uterine rupture:
    - spontaneous labour: 1 in 200
    - induction of labour at 37-40 weeks: 1 in 200
    - induction of labour after 40 weeks: 3 in 100
    - augmentation with oxytocin: 2 in 100
    - inter-delivery interval of less than 18 months: 5 in 100
        - any previous vaginal birth is associated with a reduced risk
    - multiple pregnancy – the risk of rupture is no higher than with a singleton pregnancy
        - the risk of rupture does not increase for women awaiting spontaneous onset of labour after 40 weeks (in the absence of other risk factors)
            - the early diagnosis of uterine rupture is crucial and is suggested if:
                - there is a sudden onset of an abnormal FHR pattern
                - she complains of severe abdominal pain especially in between contractions
                - there is acute onset of scar tenderness or fresh vaginal bleeding
                - there is unexplained maternal tachycardia

        - there is a cessation of previous uterine activity

- Hypoxic ischaemic encephalopathy (HIE) – these mostly occur with uterine rupture
- Antepartum stillbirth (4/1000 compared with 2/1000 for elective repeat CS)
- Perinatal mortality (PNM) 3.2/1000 versus 1.3/1000 – mostly related to antepartum deaths after 40-41 weeks
    - same as the woman labouring for the first time
    - higher than if she is having a repeat elective caesarean section
- Perineal tears and long term pelvic organ prolapse

Risks associated with elective repeat c-section

- Complications related to the anaesthetic given for the caesarean birth
- Damage to adjacent structures
- Haemorrhage and need for blood transfusion
- Hysterectomy
- Respiratory distress in the newborn
    - transient tachypnoea of the newborn
- Fever and wound infection (1 in 10 cases)
- Longer hospital stay and longer recovery period
- Ongoing pain and discomfort around the scar
- A higher risk of developing a thromboembolism
- Maternal mortality
    - 4/100,000 with VBAC
    - 13/100,000 with an elective repeat CS
- Adhesion/scar formation – over long periods this may cause chronic pain
- Future pregnancy complications
    - a higher chance of a low lying placenta and placenta accreta
        - risk increase with each consecutive repeat CS: 0.24%, 0.3%, 0.58%, 2.1%, 2.3% and 6.8%

Benefits of a repeat elective caesarean section

- Some women believe that
    - as they know what to expect they feel this is the best and safer option for themselves and it is easier to organise the birth in advance as they know the date of the birth
- Avoiding labour and the risks associated with a vaginal birth after a caesarean section

- For some medical conditions or an overwhelming fear of childbirth which has a significant effect on their mental health, a CS may be a safer alternative
- A planned CS compared to an emergency CS is less likely to cause a haemorrhage, injuries to the bladder or bowel, or to lead to infection
- There is less chance of going into labour and then having an emergency CS

Benefits of a VBAC compared to caesarean delivery

- Avoidance of risks associated with surgery
- Avoidance of anaesthetic complications
- Lower postpartum febrile morbidity
- Lower incidence of thromboembolic disease
- A shorter hospital stay and quicker recovery
- Lower risk of developing respiratory distress in the newborn
- Many women find a vaginal birth more fulfilling

Induction of labour

- Use prostaglandins with caution in women with a previous CS (it increases the risk of a uterine rupture)
    - recommend Foley/double balloon catheters

Intrapartum management

- Recommend a critical review of the progress in labour
- Recommend continuous fetal heart monitoring
    - an abnormal FHR may be an early indicator of an impending uterine rupture
- Recommend intravenous access (use a size 16 or 18 cannula)
- Send blood for group and hold
- Augment labour with caution
- An epidural in labour is safe and does not mask signs of a rupture
    - the success rate of a VBAC is improved if she has an epidural
- Allow only clear fluids orally during labour

Use of decision aids like the one shown below are useful in allowing women to make an informed decision.

Next Birth after Caesarean Section

This clinic will aim to provide you with evidence-based and unbiased information about your choices of how to birth your baby: a vaginal birth (VBAC) or an elective repeat caesarean section (ERCS).

Both are safe. However, having a baby always involves some risk, no matter what kind of birth you have.

"Our aim is to empower you to make the right choices for you"

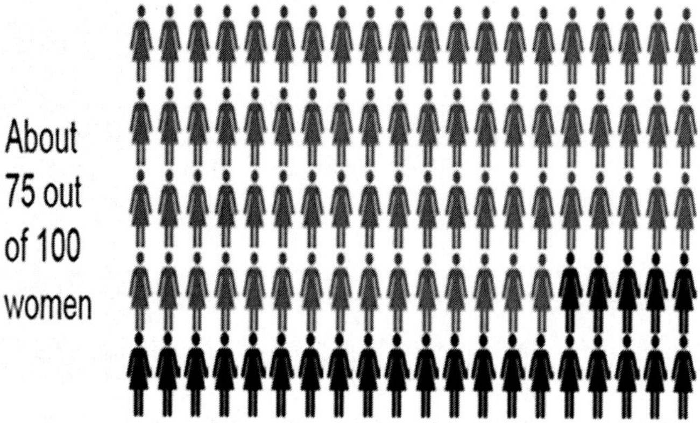

This picture shows that of all women who attempt a vaginal birth after a previous caesarean section and go into spontaneous labour, those shown in green (75 percent), will successfully give birth vaginally.

What are some of the benefits of a VBAC?

1. You avoid another scar on your uterus – **this is important**. The more caesarean sections you have the greater the chance of problems with future pregnancies – low lying placenta, placenta growing into the scar, haemorrhage, hysterectomy etc.
2. Some women believe that:
    - a vaginal birth will be a life changing experience for them
    - having a vaginal birth is the best and safest option in their situation
    - a vaginal birth will give them more control of their body.

3. With a vaginal birth there is less pain, less blood loss and less chance of infection.
4. There are no complications associated with surgery.
5. You spend fewer days in hospital and have a shorter recovery time at home.
6. There is less risk of your baby having breathing difficulties and being in the Special Care Unit.

What are some of the benefits of an ERCS?

1. Some women believe that:
    - as they know what to expect they feel this is the best and safer option for them and it is easier to organise the birth in advance as they know the date it will happen.
2. You avoid labour and the risks associated with a vaginal birth after a caesarean section.
3. For some medical conditions or due to an overwhelming fear of childbirth (which has a significant effect on mental health), a caesarean section may be a safer alternative.
4. A planned caesarean section compared to an emergency caesarean section is less likely to cause a haemorrhage, injuries to the bladder or bowel, or lead to infection.
5. There is less chance of going into labour and then having an emergency caesarean section.
6. There is a reduced risk of an unexplained stillbirth after 39 weeks.

What are some of the risks of a VBAC?

1. **Uterine rupture** – there is no way of knowing for certain who will have a uterine rupture (the scar on the uterus coming apart). The risk of uterine rupture varies according to the following:

Spontaneous labour	1 in 200
Induction of labour	1 in 100
Augmentation with Oxytocin	1 in 100
Inter-delivery interval of less than 18 months	5 in 100

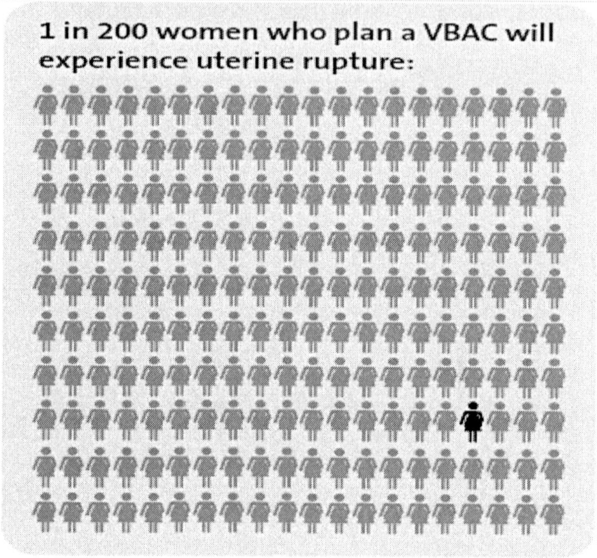

As shown in the picture, 1 in 200 women who plan a VBAC will experience uterine rupture.

2. **Damage to pelvic floor muscles** - in any vaginal birth there is always a possibility of damage to the pelvic floor muscles resulting in various types of perineal tears. This may result in pelvic organ prolapse later in life. However, pregnancy itself usually contributes to a prolapse and a caesarean section may not prevent a prolapse.
3. **Emergency caesarean section** – in some cases there may be a need for a caesarean section in labour, in which case the risks mentioned below are a bit higher.

What are some of the risks of an ERCS?

1. Like any major surgery, a caesarean section can result in surgery related problems. Examples are:
    - injury to bladder or bowel
    - haemorrhage, needing blood transfusion and rarely a hysterectomy
    - fever and wound infection (1 in 10 cases)
    - ongoing pain and discomfort around the scar
    - a higher risk of developing clots in the legs or the lungs

- adhesion/scar formation – over a long period this may cause chronic pain.

2. Complications related to the anaesthetic given for the caesarean birth.
3. A longer hospital stay and recovery period.
4. Babies born by a caesarean section may have some breathing problems as fluid is not squeezed from their lungs – most of these are mild and babies recover quickly.
5. Future pregnancy complications – an important consideration for the future:
   - With an ERCS there is a higher chance of a low-lying placenta and the placenta growing into the scar of the uterus (placenta accreta) – these can cause a severe haemorrhage with a risk of hysterectomy and, albeit rarely, can be life threatening.
6. Maternal death – the rate is 5-10/100,000 with a VBAC versus 13/100,000 with an ERCS.

Things that increase the chance of having a successful vaginal birth

- You have had a vaginal birth previously
- The reason for your previous caesarean birth is not a factor this time
- You are less than 40 years old
- You are not overweight (e.g., a BMI less than 30) or your baby weighs less than 4kg
- Your labour begins on its own and progresses normally

Things that reduce the chance of having a successful vaginal birth

- You are induced into labour
- You are 35 or older
- You have had a previous caesarean section for failure to progress in labour
- You are overweight (e.g., a BMI greater than 30) or your baby's estimated birth weight is more than 4kg

This table compares risks to you and your baby if you attempt a VBAC or an ERCS.

Likelihood of	**VBAC**	**ERCS**
1. Perineal tears	4 in 100	N/A
2. Blood transfusion	2 in 100	1 in 100
3. Serious complications in a future pregnancy	N/A if a successful VBAC	A higher risk of placenta praevia and placenta accreta
Risks to the newborn		
1. Respiratory Distress Syndrome/Transient Tachypnoea of the Newborn	2-3 in 100	4-6 in 100
2. Hypoxic brain damage	8 in 10,000	Less than 1 in 10,000
3. Stillbirth after 39 weeks	10 in 10,000	N/A
4. **If a uterine rupture occurs then it could lead to:**		
• a brain injury	3 in 10000	N/A
• the baby dying	3 in 10000	N/A
• a hysterectomy	1 in 1000	N/A

How will I be cared for if I decide to have a VBAC?

1. **Spontaneous onset of labour** - when in labour we would recommend:
    - that you come to the hospital early in labour
    - that you have an IV cannula inserted – in case we need to give you fluids or blood if there are any complications
    - your baby's heart rate will be monitored using a continuous monitoring machine – this is important as we

may be able to detect early if your baby is getting stressed possibly due to the scar opening up

- as your labour and baby's heartbeat are closely monitored we often detect a possible rupture early, however this is not always the case as sometimes it is very sudden
- regular examinations to ensure your labour is progressing satisfactorily
- in relation to pain relief in labour it is your decision whether you choose to have an epidural or not.

2. **Induction of labour** – for induction of labour we would recommend a balloon catheter to soften and open up the cervix as this is less likely to be associated with an increased risk of rupturing the uterus.

If **you had planned a repeat caesarean section** and you break your waters or present in established labour (10-15 percent chance) before the scheduled surgery **you can opt to attempt a vaginal birth if you wish** or **go ahead with the caesarean section**.

Please use this in conjunction with the information pamphlet 'Next Birth After a Caesarean Section'

Is an interpreter required? ☐ Yes ☐ No

If Yes, is a qualified interpreter present? ☐ Yes ☐ No

Please check to indicate each topic that has been discussed

☐ 'Next Birth After a Caesarean Section' pamphlet provided and discussed with the patient

☐ Previous Caesarean Section OT notes verified suitability of VBAC

If No – request for later verification

Number of months between previous CS and estimated due date: __________

☐ Risks of a VBAC

☐ Risks of an ERCS

☐ Benefits of an ERCS

☐ Factors that increase success of VBAC

☐ Benefits of a VBAC

☐ Factors that decrease success rate of VBAC

Comments

Staff Signature Log

Name (please print): ....

Designation: ....

Signature: ....

Date: _______ / ________ / ________

Please check to indicate each topic that has been discussed

If for ERCS comment on the plan if she has a Premature Rupture of Membranes (PROM) before her ERCS date:

☐ Await onset of labour and have a VBAC ☐ Have an ERCS

<table>
<tr><td colspan="3">If for ERCS comment on the plan if she comes in labour prior to her ERCS date:</td></tr>
<tr><td colspan="2">☐ She wishes to attempt VBAC</td><td>☐ She wishes to go ahead with ERCS</td></tr>
<tr><td colspan="3">If she wishes to attempt a VBAC comment on a plan if she does not go into labour by herself:</td></tr>
<tr><td>☐ She wishes to have an ERCS at 40 weeks</td><td>☐ She wishes to have an ERCS at 41 weeks</td><td>☐ She wishes to have Induction of Labour (IOL) at 41^3 and understands the risks</td></tr>
<tr><td colspan="3">Comments</td></tr>
<tr><td colspan="3"></td></tr>
</table>

Recommended Reading

1. Clarke M, Devane D, Gross MM, et al. OptiBIRTH: a cluster randomised trial of a complex intervention to increase vaginal birth after caesarean section. *BMC Pregnancy Childbirth*. 2020 Mar 6; 20(1): 143.
2. Bartolo S, Goffinet F, Blondel B et al. Why women with previous caesarean and eligible for a trial of labour have an elective repeat caesarean delivery? A national study in France. *BJOG.* 2016 Sep; 123(10): 1664-73.
3. Kuppermann M, Kaimal AJ, Blat C et al. Effect of a Patient-Centered Decision Support Tool on Rates of Trial of Labor After Previous Cesarean Delivery: The PROCEED Randomized Clinical Trial. *JAMA*. 2020 Jun 2; 323(21): 2151-2159.
4. Tanos V, Toney ZA. Uterine scar rupture - Prediction, prevention, diagnosis, and management. *Best Pract. Res. Clin. Obstet. Gynaecol.* 2019 Aug; 59: 115-131.
5. Lundgren I, Healy P, Carroll M et al. Clinicians' views of factors of importance for improving the rate of VBAC (vaginal birth after

caesarean section): a study from countries with low VBAC rates. *BMC Pregnancy Childbirth.* 2016 Nov 10; 16(1): 350.

6. American College of Obstetricians and Gynecologists' Committee on Practice Bulletins—Obstetrics. ACOG Practice Bulletin No. 205: Vaginal Birth After Cesarean Delivery. *Obstet. Gynecol.* 2019 Feb; 133(2): e110-e127.
7. Vankan E, Schoorel E, van Kuijk S et al. The effect of the use of a decision aid with individual risk estimation on the mode of delivery after a caesarean section: A prospective cohort study. Nijhuis J, Hermens R, Scheepers H; SIMPLE study group.
8. Martel MJ, MacKinnon CJ. No. 155 - Guidelines for Vaginal Birth After Previous Caesarean Birth. *Obstet. Gynaecol. Can.* 2018 Mar; 40(3): e195-e207.
9. Sentilhes et al. Delivery for women with a previous cesarean: guidelines for clinical practice from the French College of Gynecologists and Obstetricians (CNGOF) / *European Journal of Obstetrics & Gynecology and Reproductive Biology.* 170 (2013); 5–32.
10. Harris BS, Heine RP, Park J et al. Are prediction models for vaginal birth after cesarean accurate? *Am. J. Obstet. Gynecol.* 2019 May; 220(5): 492.e1-492.e7.

CHAPTER SIXTY-SIX

VAGINAL BIRTH AFTER MORE THAN ONE PREVIOUS CAESAREAN SECTION (VBAC-2/3)

Obstetricians generally prefer a third planned caesarean section (CS) in women with two previous CSs, partly based on:

- Large overestimation of immediate maternal and neonatal serious outcomes associated with a trial of labour
- Insufficient consideration of serious long-term outcomes associated with multiple caesarean sections

Women requesting a vaginal birth are generally not allowed or counselled appropriately and may receive conflicting advice, an issue likely to be of considerable importance to many women

- A 2010 paper concluded that women with three or more prior CSs who attempted a vaginal birth had similar rates of success and risks for maternal morbidity as those with one prior CS, similar to women who have an elective repeat CS
- Two recent studies have noted that if one follows a strict protocol, trial of labour after two previous CSs can be a reasonable alternative and is associated with favourable outcomes
- The ACOG Practice Bulletin states that it is "reasonable to consider" a trial of labour in women with two previous caesarean sections

There are no RCTs to guide clinicians on how best to discuss this topic

- A systematic review of mostly cohort studies including 5,666 women undergoing labour (mostly as planned trial of labour) after two or more CSs showed:
    - success rates for a VBAC-2 were 71.1% versus 76.5% for a VBAC -1
    - uterine rupture rates for a VBAC-2 were 1.59% versus 0.72% for VBAC- 1
        - the risk was lower with history of prior vaginal delivery

        - the risk is higher with induction or augmentation in labour
            - if there is a uterine rupture, perinatal mortality is 3-6% and neonatal asphyxia (umbilical artery pH < 7.00 or neonatal encephalopathy) is 6-15%

    - women requiring a blood transfusion for VBAC-2 was 1.99% versus 1.21% for VBAC-1
    - febrile morbidity for VBAC-2 was 6.03% versus 6.39% for VBAC-1
    - neonatal asphyxial injury/perinatal death (attributable to mode of delivery) rates were similar for VBAC-1 and VBAC-2
        - a recent review however suggested an increase odds ratio of 1.78 in severe neonatal complications
- Counsel women requesting to have a trial of vaginal birth after two caesarean sections appropriately considering the available evidence
- Clearly document the care plan
- An ultrasound scan to measure scar thickness may be useful
    - some reports suggest having a thickness of the lower uterine segment of 3.5mm or more on an ultrasound scan at 38 weeks is a good sign
    - a thickness of < 1.8mm would indicate a very thin lower segment and an indication to avoid vaginal birth

Induction of labour (IOL)

- Avoid IOL unless the cervical Bishop score is 6 or more, in which case a sweep and stretch and Atad catheter may be used

Intrapartum management

- Monitor the progress of labour strictly
- Recommend continuous fetal heart monitoring
- See the chapter on VBAC-1

Cessation of VBAC-2 or VBAC-3

- Stagnation of cervical dilatation over more than 2 hours in the active phase of labour
- If there is **any** fetal heart rate abnormality

Recommended Reading

1. Tahseen S, Griffiths M. Vaginal birth after two caesarean sections (VBAC-2) - a systematic review with meta-analysis of success rate and adverse outcomes of VBAC-2 versus VBAC-1 and repeat (third) caesarean sections. *BJOG*. 2010 Jan; 117(1): 5-19.
2. Davidson C, Bellows P, Shah U et al. Outcomes associated with trial of labor after cesarean in women with one versus two prior cesarean deliveries after a change in clinical practice guidelines in an academic hospital. *J. Mat. Fetal Neonatal Med*. 2020 May; 33(9): 1499-1504.
3. Rotem R, Hirsch A, Sela HY et al. Maternal and Neonatal Outcomes Following Trial of Labor After Two Previous Cesareans: a Retrospective Cohort Study. *Reprod. Sci.* 2020 Nov 13. doi: 10.1007/s43032-020-00378-1.
4. De Leo R, La Gamba DA, Manzoni P Vaginal Birth after Two Previous Cesarean Sections versus Elective Repeated Cesarean: A Retrospective Study. *Am. J. Perinatol*. 2020 Sep; 37(S 02): S84-S88.
5. Dombrowski M, Illuzzi JL, Reddy UM et al. Trial of Labor After Two Prior Cesarean Deliveries: Patient and Hospital Characteristics and Birth Outcomes. *Obstet. Gynecol*. 2020 Jul; 136(1): 109-117.

CHAPTER SIXTY-SEVEN

VASA PRAEVIA

Fetal vessels course through membranes overlying the internal os ahead of the presenting part.

- This is often an incidental finding on a scan
  - it may present with a fresh painless vaginal bleed
- It is more common with IVF pregnancies
- Risk factors include placenta praevia and multiple pregnancy
- If the vessel ruptures it may lead to fetal exsanguination
- Two major risk factors for vasa praevia are velamentous insertion of the cord (which accounts for the majority of cases) and succenturiate lobe or a bilobed placenta

Risk factors include

Approximately 60% of women with vasa praevia at delivery have a placenta praevia or low lying placenta identified during the second-trimester ultrasound scan

- It is associated with velamentous insertion of the cord or a separate succenturiate lobe
  - in such cases monitor the fetal growth
- In vitro fertilization
- Increased prevalence of vasa praevia with multiple pregnancy

If a woman with vasa praevia presents with active bleeding

  - consider doing a bed side Apt test (add 2-3 drops of concentrated alkaline solution like KOH to 1ml of vaginal blood; the maternal blood will turn brown, the fetal blood will remain red
  - recommend an urgent MCA doppler velocity

Diagnosis

- Maternal and fetal outcomes are significantly improved when vasa previa has been diagnosed antenatally
- It is usually seen during the morphology scan
    - o 20% of these cases will resolve spontaneously before labour
- Recommend a repeat scan at a tertiary centre

Management

- Recommend antenatal corticosteroids at 32 weeks of gestation in case of the need for urgent preterm delivery
- Consider hospitalisation at 30-34 weeks of gestation
- Deliver before the rupture of the membranes while minimizing the impact of iatrogenic prematurity
- Recommend a planned caesarean section for a prenatal diagnosis of vasa praevia at 34-36 weeks of gestation
    - o if the fetal vessel has been lacerated inadvertently during delivery, immediately clamp the cord to prevent fetal/neonatal blood loss
    - o aim to have immediate availability of type O negative blood, in case of the delivery of a severely anaemic neonate
- Fetal mortality > 75% especially if there has been vaginal bleeding

Recommended Reading

1. Gagnon R. Guidelines for the Management of Vasa Previa. No 21. *J. Obstet. Gynaecol. Can.* 2017 Oct; 39(10): e415-e421.
2. Swank ML, Garite TJ, Maurel K et al. Vasa preavia diagnosis and management. Obstetric Collaborative Research Network. *Am. J. Obstet. Gynecol.* 2016 Aug; 215(2): 223.
3. Sinkey RG, Odibo AO, Dashe JS Diagnosis and management of vasa previa. Society of Maternal-Fetal (SMFM) Publications Committee. *Am. J. Obstet. Gynecol.* 2015 Nov; 213(5): 615-9.
4. Ranzini AC, Oyelese Y. How to screen for vasa previa. *Ultrasound Obstet. Gynecol.* 2021 May; 57(5): 720-725.
5. Zhang W, Geris S, Beta J et al. Prevention of stillbirth: impact of two-stage screening for vasa previa. *Ultrasound Obstet Gynecol.* 2020 May; 55(5): 605-612.

6. Jauniaux E, Alfirevic Z, Bhide AG et al. Royal College of Obstetricians and Gynaecologists. Vasa Praevia: Diagnosis and Management: Green-top Guideline No. 27b. *BJOG*. 2019 Jan; 126(1): e49-e61.

CHAPTER SIXTY-EIGHT

VENOUS THROMBOEMBOLISM – PREVENTION

Incidence: It occurs in 1-2 per 1,000 pregnancies and it is the second most common cause of direct maternal death – pulmonary embolism has a higher maternal mortality rate.

Risk factors for venous thromboembolism (VTE)

High risk factors:
- Personal history of unprovoked VTE before or during any previous pregnancy or the current one
- Recurrent provoked VTE
- Thrombophilia and a family history of VTE in a first degree relative
- Medical comorbidity – cardiac failure, active SLE, sickle cell anaemia (SCA), nephrotic syndrome, active inflammatory conditions (inflammatory polyarthropathy and inflammatory bowel disease), insulin dependent diabetes with nephropathy

Other risk factors
- Socio-demographic
    - age > 35 years
    - BMI ≥ 30
    - smoking > 10 cigarettes per day
    - parity ≥ 3
- Medical
    - personal history of provoked VTE
    - FH of VTE in a first degree relative
    - antiphospholipid syndrome
    - ovarian hyper stimulation
    - pre-existing diabetes
    - previous VTE
    - inherited thrombophilia

- Pregnancy related
    - immobility
    - hyperemesis gravidarum
    - pre-eclampsia
    - assisted reproductive therapy
    - gestational diabetes
    - multiple pregnancy
    - fetal growth restriction
    - surgery in pregnancy
    - gross varicose veins
- Birth and postpartum
    - prolonged labour > 24 hours
    - caesarean section
    - operative vaginal birth
    - postpartum haemorrhage (> 1litre) requiring blood transfusion
    - postpartum infection

The most common risk factors that have been identified include: hospitalization (10.4%), previous surgery (10.4%) and a family history of VTE.

Prevention of VTE in pregnancy

The template below gives guidance to indications for thromboprophylaxis antenatally and postpartum.

- Perform a risk assessment at a booking in visit and at 28 and 34 weeks (at least)
- Low molecular weight heparin (LMWH) is the drug of choice
- Timing and dosage are as per the template below
- The dose of LMWH is based on BMI
- There is no need to monitor the platelet count if a woman has had prior exposure to unfractionated Heparin (UFH)
- There is no need for routine monitoring of anti-Xa levels with the use of LMWH
- LMWH is safe in breastfeeding
- Unfractionated Heparin may be used peripartum in preference to LMWH when there is a higher risk of bleeding or if one anticipates the need for an epidural or spinal
    - if UFH is used, monitor her platelet count every 2-3 days from days 4-14 or until Heparin is stopped

1. Labour and birth management – on therapeutic anticoagulation

- Plan the delivery beforehand – induction of labour (IOL) or caesarean section (CS)
- Use TEDS stockings and intermittent calf compression and encourage early mobilisation
- Stop LMWH and initiate intravenous unfractionated Heparin 24-36 hours before any elective procedure
- If an epidural is not safe, recommend an intravenous patient-controlled analgesia with opiates

Induction of labour

- Stop intravenous Heparin as soon as labour is established
- Manage labour as normal, encouraging mobility
- Recommend active management of the third stage

Caesarean section

- For an emergency CS with prolonged APTT – administer fresh frozen plasma
- For an elective CS stop intravenous unfractionated Heparin 6 hours before the procedure

Regional anaesthesia/analgesia considerations

- These are contraindicated during anticoagulation treatment
- Cease all anticoagulant treatment at least 24 hours before any regional anaesthesia or planned elective CS
- Keep the epidural catheter in place for 12 hours after the last therapeutic anticoagulant dose
- Delay the next anticoagulant intravenous/subcutaneous injection for 6 hours following the removal of the epidural catheter
- Monitor for signs or symptoms of spinal haematoma (lower limb numbness or weakness, severe back pain, urinary or faecal incontinence)

2. Labour and birth management – on prophylactic anticoagulation

- Advice that anticoagulants be ceased if she shows any symptoms of labour
- For elective CS
    - omit the morning dose of LMWH
        - restart 6 hours after the CS or after catheter removal
- For IOL
    - have the morning dose of LMWH
    - cease further until after birth
- If an epidural is not safe, recommend intravenous patient-controlled analgesia with opiates
- Delay the next anticoagulant intravenous/subcutaneous injection for 6 hours following removal of the epidural catheter.

Breast feeding

- This is safe with LMWH, Heparin or Warfarin.

HIGH RISK

1. Assess each woman individually for VTE
2. Assess at: (a) booking in visit and subsequent antenatal visits; (b) any Antenatal admission; and (c) Postnatal period
3. If unsure discuss with the Registrar/Consultant
4. Discuss options for VTE prophylaxis with the woman
5. Document a plan of care

1. Any woman on antenatal thromboprophylaxis needs to continue same for 6 weeks postpartum (PP)

2. Pre-existing High Risk Factor – Therapeutic Clexane antenatally (the form of anticoagulation may need to be modified – seek physician advice)

- ☐ Previous VTE on long term anticoagulation
- ☐ On long term anticoagulation for any reason
- ☐ Previous VTE plus (antiphospholipid syndrome) or (antithrombin def)
- ☐ Recurrent unprovoked VTE
- ☐ VTE in current pregnancy

3. Thomboprophylaxis – 40mg Clexane (60mg if BMI ≥ 40)

- ☐ Any Hospital admission > 3 days – while in hospital
- ☐ Ovarian Hyper-stimulation Syndrome – for the first trimester
- ☐ Any surgery in pregnancy or postpartum – while in hospital
- ☐ Hyperemesis – from admission until it resolves

4. High Risk Factor – Antenatal Clexane 40mg daily and continue for 6 weeks postpartum

- ☐ Previous VTE not related to surgery
- ☐ High Risk thrombophilia (antithrombin def, Protein S, C def, homozygous factor V gene mutation, combination of low risk thrombophilia
- ☐ Recurrent provoked VTE
- ☐ Medical comorbidity (Congestive Cardiac Failure, active Systemic Lupus Erythematosus, active inflammatory polyarthropathy, Nephrotic syndrome, Insulin Dependent Diabetes with nephropathy, Sickle Cell Anaemia)

ALL RISK

5. ANTENATAL		6. POSTNATAL	
Add Antenatal and Postpartum Scores			
Score ≤ 2:	Early Mobilisation, avoid dehydration	**Score < 1:**	Early mobilisation, avoid dehydration and discuss Graduated Compression Stockings for up to 14 days
Score 3:	A/N Thromboprophylaxis from 28 weeks	**Score 2:**	Above +40mg Clexane until discharge
Score ≥ 4:	A/N Thromboprophylaxis	**Score > 3:**	Above +40mg for 7 days
			***Commence Clexane within 6hrs of birth - 60mg if BMI ≥ 40** ***All Caesarean Sections – recommend Sequential Compression Devices until the next day**

Antenatal Scores				**Postnatal Score**	
☐ Age > 35	1	☐ Family History of VTE in 1st degree relative unrelated to surgery	1	☐ Prolonged labour ≥ 18 hrs	1
☐ Parity ≥ 3	1	☐ IVF Pregnancy	1	☐ PPH (>1 litre/transfusion)	1
☐ BMI > 30	1	☐ Multiple Pregnancy	1	☐ Non lift out operative vaginal delivery	1
☐ BMI > 40	2	☐ Gross varicose veins	1	☐ Admission for PP endometritis	1
☐ Smoking > 10/day	1	☐ Current Systemic Infection	1	☐ Elective caesarean section	2
☐ Heterozygous Factor V leiden	1	☐ Pre-Eclampsia	1	☐ Caesarean section in labour	3
☐ Heterozygous Prothrombin gene mutation	1	☐ Immobility	1	☐ Stillbirth	1
☐ Anti phospholipid antibodies	1			☐ Preterm birth <37 weeks	1
☐ Pre-existing Diabetes	1			☐ Caesarean hysterectomy	3
☐ Single VTE Provoked by surgery	3				

Date	Gestation	AN Score	Action	Signature	Date	Total AN/PN Score	Action	Signature

Signature Log

Name (please print):... Designation:...

Signature:... Date: ____/__ __/______

Recommended Reading

1. Gonik B, editors. *High risk pregnancy: management options*, 5th ed. London: Harcourt; 2017, pp. 753-62.
2. Tromeura C. et al. Pitfalls in the diagnostic management of pulmonary embolism in pregnancy. Thrombosis Research 2017; 151: Suppl. 1 S86–S91.
3. Royal College of Obstetrics and Gynaecology (RCOG). Clinical Green Top Guidelines - Reducing the risk of thromboembolism during pregnancy and the puerperium (37a): April 2015.
4. Middleton P, Shepherd E, Gomersall JC. Venous thromboembolism prophylaxis for women at risk during pregnancy and the early postnatal period. *Cochrane Database Syst. Rev*. 2021 Mar 29; 3(3): CD001689.
5. Kearsley R, Stocks G. Venous thromboembolism in pregnancy-diagnosis, management, and treatment. *BJA Educ.* 2021 Mar; 21(3): 117-123.
6. Xu L, Zhang Y, Wang Z, Gao C, Yu Q, Zhang L. Clinical study of heparin combined with aspirin in the treatment of thromboembolism and its effect on pregnancy outcomes. *Minerva Med.* 2021 Feb 8. doi: 10.23736/S0026-4806.20.07236-5.
7. Bates SM. Pulmonary Embolism in Pregnancy. *Semin. Respir. Crit. Care Med.* 2021 Apr; 42(2): 284-298.
8. Shirazi M, Sahebdel B, Torkzaban M, Feizabad E, Ghaemi M. Maternal mortality following thromboembolism; incidences and prophylaxis strategies. *Thromb. J.* 2020 Nov 30; 18(1): 36.
9. Friedman AM, D'Alton M. Society for Maternal-Fetal Medicine Consult Series #51: thromboembolism prophylaxis for cesarean delivery. *Am. J. Obstet. Gynecol.* 2021 Feb; 224(2): 243-244.
10. Nicholson M, Chan N, Bhagirath V, Ginsberg J. Prevention of Venous Thromboembolism in 2020 and Beyond. *J. Clin. Med.* 2020 Aug 1; 9(8): 2467. doi: 10.3390/jcm9082467.
11. O'Shaughnessy F, O'Reilly D, Ní Áinle F. Current opinion and emerging trends on the treatment, diagnosis, and prevention of pregnancy-associated venous thromboembolic disease: a review. *Transl. Res.* 2020 Nov; 225: 20-32.

CHAPTER SIXTY-NINE

VENOUS THROMBOEMBOLISM – DIAGNOSIS AND MANAGEMENT

- Signs and symptoms of deep vein thrombosis (DVT), pulmonary embolism (PE) and cerebral vein thrombosis (CVT) overlap with normal pregnancy-related physiologic changes
- There is swelling of the legs
- There is abdominal pain if she has pelvic vein thrombosis
- There is lack of a validated test for use in pregnancy (D-dimer assays cannot be relied on)
    - symptoms in the left leg, calf circumference difference > 2cm, and first trimester presentation are good indications for imaging for DVT in pregnant women
- Concern over radiation exposure:
    - fetal radiation exposure is many times less than the dose that would cause pregnancy loss and/or fetal malformations
        - there is a small absolute increase in the risk of childhood cancer

Deep vein thrombosis

Clinical features of DVT- use these and risk factors in combination to avoid missing a diagnosis

- Previous history
- Known thrombophilia
- High BMI
- Smoking
- IVF pregnancy
- Multiple pregnancy
- 90% of deep venous thromboses in pregnant women occur in the left leg
- Mostly they affect proximal veins – iliofemoral is much more common than calf veins

- It is almost always unilateral
- Unilateral leg pain, may be associated with swelling
- Increased temperature over the area
- Homans' sign may be positive

Confirm diagnosis: This is important as it has implications for long term anticoagulation, management of the current and any future pregnancy and an effect on the type of contraception to be recommended

- Doppler ultrasound scan – proximal vein with a colour Doppler as the initial test
    - do a 2-point scan of the common femoral vein at the groin and the popliteal vein at the popliteal fossa
- If you suspect iliac vein DVT, carry out doppler ultrasonography of the iliac vein, venography, or magnetic resonance imaging
    - suspect it if there's swelling of the whole leg with back, buttock or flank pain
- In women with suspected DVT, if you're initially uncertain withhold treatment and rescan after 2-3 days
- D-dimers are increased with DVT, but these are normally raised during pregnancy and increase dramatically postpartum; testing is shown to be of value to safely rule out VTE in pregnant women with suspected VTE

Complications from DVT

- Pulmonary embolism
- Maternal mortality
- Postphlebitic limb syndrome (swelling, pain and ulceration)
- Risks associated with treatment (heparin – osteoporosis) and thrombocytopenia

Pulmonary Embolism

- It often occurs when risk factors for venous thromboembolism (VTE) are not recognised and adequate prophylaxis is not commenced
- Obvious clinical features may not always be present
    - fever, cough or pleuritic chest pain, shortness of breath

Diagnosis

- An electrocardiogram is often performed but it is insensitive and very nonspecific
- Do blood gases to assess hypoxia but this is usually normal

- If the woman presents with signs and symptoms of lower extremity deep vein thrombosis (DVT)
    - request a doppler scan as the first line (as above)
        - if consistent with a DVT, assume diagnosis of PE in the presence of chest symptoms
        - no further imaging is needed, as treatment is the same for DVT and PE
- If there are no clinical features of DVT and suspect PE, proceed directly to exclude PE and avoid doing a scan of the lower limbs
    - recommend an urgent chest x-ray with shielding the fetus – may show a cause for the symptoms, such as pneumothorax or pneumonia
    - if CXR is abnormal, request a CTPA
    - if CXR is normal, request a V/Q scan
        - radiation dose from CTPA or V-Q lung scanning are both well below the threshold for fetal radiation complications
            - with a V/Q scan, the risk of fatal childhood cancer is 1/17,000
        - a CTPA results in considerably higher total body maternal radiation, with particularly high doses to maternal breast tissue
        - a V/Q scan has a higher fetal radiation exposure – to avoid radiation exposure, perform a perfusion scan first and if its results are abnormal proceed with a ventilation scan
            - choice of which test to do first depends on the clinician, radiologist and the rapid availability of the test
            - an MRI may be used to confirm but not for the initial diagnosis – the exposure risk to the fetus is uncertain
- If you suspect pelvic DVT, the gravid uterus may obscure imaging and further evaluation with magnetic resonance imaging (MRI) may be required

Cerebral vein thrombosis (CVT)

- The reported frequency of CVT in pregnancy and the puerperium is 12 cases per 100,000
    - it occurs mostly in the third trimester and postpartum

Clinical features

- 90% of women will have a headache, usually building up over days, but may also be severe with acute onset
- They may also have vomiting, papilledema, visual changes, and focal neurologic features including seizures

Diagnosis

- Use non contrast medical resistance venography (MRV) with an MRI as the first-line imaging test

Management of VTE in pregnancy - prompt therapeutic anticoagulation

- Tests prior to commencing therapy include activated partial thromboplastin time or aPTT (if it's raised suspect lupus anticoagulant); an FBC; a thrombophilia screen; and urea, electrolytes and liver-function tests
    - LMWH is the preferred first line drug – prescribe Enoxaparin (Clexane) 1mg/kg subcutaneously twice daily
        - it's highly efficacious with a low risk of bleeding complications
        - there's a negligible risk of Heparin-induced thrombocytopenia (HIT) and osteoporosis
        - it has better bioavailability
        - it has a longer plasma half-life
        - it has a more predictable dose response
        - there's no need to monitor drug activity in most situations
        - it does not cross the placenta and thus is not associated with fetal complications, and is safe to use in breastfeeding women
    - UFH can also be used (usually administered intravenously by continuous infusion) – the dose is adjusted to achieve therapeutic aPTT
        - the dosing is weight-based
        - the recommended regimen is 5,000 units bolus followed by 100 units per hour for 1 week and then maintenance therapy (10,000 units subcutaneously

twice daily or change to LMWH (Clexane 40mg subcutaneously daily)
        - monitor the adequacy of anticoagulation with aPTT testing 4-6 hours after the initial dose and then daily and maintain it to 1.5 to 2 times control
        - monitoring of anti-Xa levels is not recommended
        - ACOG recommends twice daily dosing
    - Warfarin is teratogenic between 6 and 12 weeks of gestation, and is associated with fetal and neonatal bleeding complications
        - it is generally avoided in pregnancy
        - it is however preferred in pregnant women with mechanical heart valves

Side effects of anticoagulation

- Osteoporosis – exposure of > 3 months. It is less likely to occur with LMWH than with UFH
- Heparin induced thrombocytopaenia (HIT) occurs with UFH mostly but can occur with therapeutic doses of LMWH; the platelet count drops around days 5-10 and in many cases the woman develops new or worsening thrombosis
    - monitor her platelet count at the onset of treatment and repeat weekly for 3 weeks
    - if she gets HIT, cease immediately and use an alternative drug

Heparin Antidote

- Protamine Sulphate
    - if < 8 hours prior to Heparin, use 1mg Protamine /100 units Heparin
    - if 8 hours or longer, use 0.5mg Protamine /100 units Heparin

Duration of anticoagulation

- For calf vein thrombosis, 6 weeks
- For DVT, 6 months
- For recurrent thromboembolism, 6 months

Labour and birth management – on therapeutic anticoagulation

- Plan delivery beforehand – IOL or CS
- Use TEDS stockings and intermittent calf compression and encourage early mobilisation
- Stop LMWH and initiate intravenous unfractionated Heparin 24-36 hours before any elective procedure

- If an epidural is not safe, use intravenous patient controlled analgesia with opiates

Induction of labour
- Stop intravenous Heparin as soon as labour is established
- Manage labour as normal and encouraging mobility
- Recommend active management of the third stage

Caesarean section
- For emergency CS with prolonged APTT – administer fresh frozen plasma
- For elective CS stop intravenous unfractionated Heparin 6 hours before

Regional anaesthesia/analgesia considerations
- These are contraindicated during anticoagulation treatment
- Cease all anticoagulant treatment at least 24 hours before any regional anaesthesia or planned elective caesarean section
- The epidural catheter should remain in place for 12 hours after the last therapeutic anticoagulant dose
- Delay the next anticoagulant intravenous/subcutaneous injection for 6 hours following removal of the epidural catheter
- Monitor for signs or symptoms of spinal haematoma (e.g., lower limb numbness or weakness, severe back pain, or urinary/faecal incontinence)

Aspirin
- There is no place for its use in the treatment of VTE

Breastfeeding
- This is safe with either Heparin or Warfarin

Contraception
- Combined oral contraceptive preparations are contraindicated

Recommended Reading

1. Tromeura C. Pitfalls in the diagnostic management of pulmonary embolism in pregnancy. *Thrombosis Research*. 2017; 151: Suppl. 1 S86–S91.
2. Royal College of Obstetrics and Gynaecology (RCOG). Clinical Green Top Guidelines - Reducing the risk of thromboembolism during pregnancy and the puerperium (37a): April 2015.
3. Bellesini M, Robert-Ebadi H, Combescure C et al. D-Dimer to rule out venous thromboembolism during pregnancy: a systematic review and meta-analysis. *J. Thromb. Haemost*. 2021 Jun 23. doi: 10.1111/jth.15432.
4. Kearsley R, Stocks G. Venous thromboembolism in pregnancy-diagnosis, management, and treatment. *BJA Educ*. 2021 Mar; 21(3): 117-123.
5. Bates SM. Pulmonary Embolism in Pregnancy. *Semin. Respir. Crit. Care Med*. 2021 Apr; 42(2): 284-298.
6. Liederman Z, Chan N, Bhagirath V. Current Challenges in Diagnosis of Venous Thromboembolism. *J. Clin. Med*. 2020 Oct 29; 9(11): 3509.
7. Duffett L, Castellucci LA, Forgie MA. Pulmonary embolism: update on management and controversies. *BMJ*. 2020 Aug 5; 370: m2177. doi: 10.1136/bmj.m2177.
8. O'Shaughnessy F, O'Reilly D, Ní Áinle F. Current opinion and emerging trends on the treatment, diagnosis, and prevention of pregnancy-associated venous thromboembolic disease: a review. *Transl. Res*. 2020 Nov; 225: 20-32.
9. Patel H, Sun H, Hussain AN, Vakde T. Advances in the Diagnosis of Venous Thromboembolism: A Literature Review. *Diagnostics* (Basel). 2020 Jun 2; 10(6): 365.
10. Wiegers HMG, Middeldorp S. Contemporary best practice in the management of pulmonary embolism during pregnancy. *Ther. Adv. Respir. Dis*. 2020 Jan-Dec; 14: 1753466620914222.